TOXIC MOLD HEALING BIBLE

A Step-by-Step Guide to Mold Toxicity, Lyme Disease, and Chronic Illness with Proven Protocols to Detox, Heal, and Restore Your Vitality

Arden Harper

© 2024 Toxic Mold Healing Bible All rights reserved. This document is designed purely for informational purposes and pertains exclusively to this book. Any unauthorized copying, sharing, or dissemination of this book, either in full or in sections, is strictly forbidden. All trademarks and brand names that appear are owned by their respective companies. The publisher does not accept any liability for any harm or damages that may arise from the application or misapplication of the information presented in this book. The book is offered 'as is,' with no guarantees, whether explicit or implied.

TABLE OF CONTENT

Part 1: Toxic Mold and Chronic Illness 7

Chapter 1: Why Mold Toxicity Matters 8

    1.1: The Hidden Dangers of Mold Exposure 11

    1.2: Mold's Impact on Body and Mind 12

    1.3: Mold, Lyme Disease, and Chronic Illness Connection 14

    1.4: Who This Book Is For 16

Chapter 2: Identifying Mold Toxicity 18

    2.1: Common Symptoms of Mold Exposure 22

    2.2: Chronic Illness or Mold Toxicity? 23

    2.3: Genetics and Mold Sensitivity 25

    2.4: Mold Toxicity Self-Assessment 27

Chapter 3: The Science of Mold Toxicity 30

    3.1: What Is Mold and Where It Thrives 30

    3.2: Mycotoxins and Their Health Impact 32

    3.3: The Cell Danger Response 33

Part 2: Diagnosing Mold Exposure 37

Chapter 4: Medical Testing for Mold Illnesses 38

    4.1: Key Medical Tests for Mold Toxicity 38

    4.2: Testing for Mycotoxins 40

    4.3: Diagnosing Lyme and Co-Infections 41

Chapter 5: Testing Your Environment 44

    5.1: Detecting Mold in Your Home 44

    5.2: Professional vs. DIY Mold Testing 45

5.3: Interpreting Test Results...47

Part 3: Protocols to Detox and Heal 49

Chapter 6: Creating a Mold-Free Environment 50

6.1: Immediate Steps to Reduce Mold Exposure 50

6.2: DIY Mold Remediation Guide...52

6.3: Hiring Mold Remediation Professionals 54

6.4: Preventing Mold Regrowth 56

Chapter 7: Detoxing Your Body...58

7.1: Supporting Liver and Detox Pathways 61

7.2: Nutritional Strategies for Detoxification 62

7.3: Key Supplements and Herbs for Mold Recovery 64

7.4: Sauna and Sweating for Detox 66

Chapter 8: Healing Your Systems 68

8.1: Rebooting Your Nervous System...71

8.2: Restoring Immune Balance 73

8.3: Repairing Gut Health After Mold Exposure 74

8.4: Managing Hormonal and Endocrine Disruptions..76

Part 4: Co-Infections and Chronic Illness..79

Chapter 9: Lyme Disease and Mold Toxicity... 80

9.1: Mold and Lyme Symptom Overlap 80

9.2: Treating Lyme and Mold Toxicity Together 82

9.3 Managing Co-Infections: Bartonella, Babesia 84

Chapter 10: Chronic Illness and Mold 86

10.1: Mold and Autoimmune Disorders..86

10.2: Mold's Role in Chronic Fatigue and Fibromyalgia..88

10.3: Supporting Long-Term Recovery 90

Part 5: Restoring Vitality and Preventing Relapse 93

Chapter 11: Emotional and Mental Healing 94

11.1: Coping with Stress and Anxiety 94

11.2: Reclaiming Emotional Balance 96

11.3: Overcoming Chronic Illness Isolation 97

Chapter 12: Rebuilding Energy and Vitality 100

12.1: Nutritional Strategies to Regain Energy 100

12.2: Gentle Exercise for Recovery 101

12.3: Sleep Optimization for Restful Nights 103

Chapter 13: Preventing Future Mold Exposure 106

13.1: Identifying High-Risk Environments 106

13.2: Building a Mold-Resistant Home 107

13.3: Lifestyle Habits for Long-Term Health 109

Resources and Appendices 111

Appendix A: DIY Mold Testing Checklist 111

Appendix B: Supplement and Herb Guide 112

Part 1:
Toxic Mold and Chronic Illness

Chapter 1: Why Mold Toxicity Matters

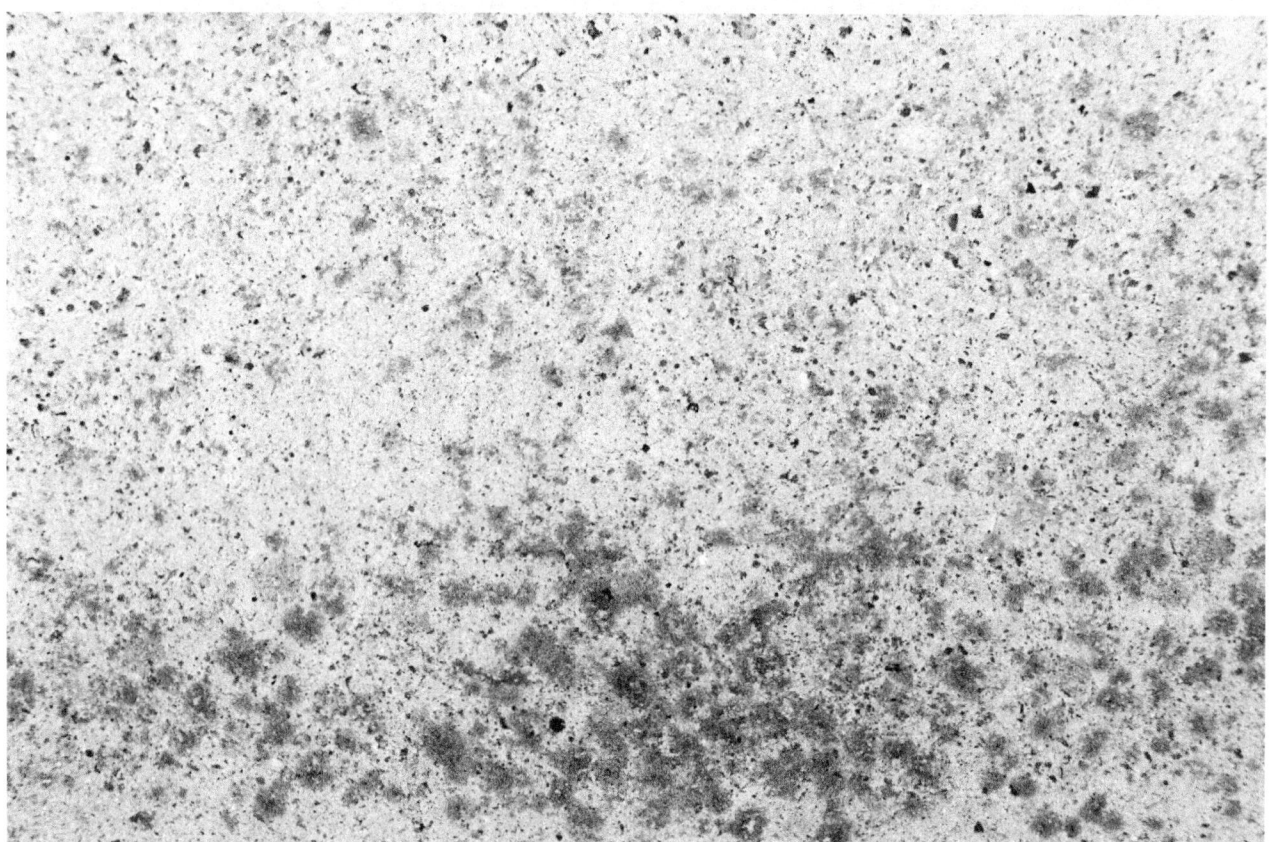

Mold toxicity, often overlooked in the medical community, represents a significant health threat that can silently infiltrate our lives, manifesting through a wide array of symptoms that mimic other illnesses. This insidious nature makes it a formidable opponent in the quest for health, as it can reside undetected in homes, workplaces, and schools, releasing harmful mycotoxins into the air we breathe. These mycotoxins are potent chemicals capable of causing a range of physical and mental health issues, from respiratory problems to cognitive dysfunction, often leading individuals down a path of misdiagnosis and ineffective treatments.

Understanding the impact of mold exposure requires a deep dive into the biological mechanisms at play. When inhaled or ingested, mycotoxins can disrupt cellular processes, leading to an immune response that, while intended to protect, can result in chronic inflammation and a host of systemic issues. This response is not uniform across all individuals, which complicates the clinical picture further. Genetic predispositions can make certain people more susceptible to mold-related illnesses, highlighting the need for personalized approaches in diagnosis and treatment.

The connection between mold exposure and chronic illness is a critical area of concern. Conditions such as Chronic Inflammatory Response Syndrome (CIRS) are directly linked to environmental factors like mold, yet the awareness and understanding of this connection are still emerging. This gap in knowledge underscores the importance of educating both the public and healthcare professionals about the signs of mold toxicity and the necessity for comprehensive environmental assessments in the management of chronic illnesses.

Moreover, the overlap of symptoms between mold toxicity and other conditions, such as Lyme disease, adds another layer of complexity to diagnosis and treatment. Both conditions can present with fatigue, brain fog, and joint pain, making it challenging to distinguish one from the other without thorough medical evaluation. This similarity can lead to a cycle of suffering for those affected, as they search for answers in a medical system that may not be equipped to consider environmental factors as a root cause of their symptoms.

As we delve further into the intricacies of mold toxicity, it becomes clear that a multifaceted approach is required to effectively address this issue. From identifying the presence of mold in one's environment to understanding the biological impact of mycotoxin exposure, each step is crucial in the journey toward recovery. The following sections will explore the scientific underpinnings of mold-related illnesses, offering insights into the latest research and practical strategies for those seeking to reclaim their health from the clutches of mold toxicity.

The role of environmental assessments cannot be overstated in the battle against mold toxicity. These evaluations are essential for uncovering hidden mold infestations that may not be immediately visible but are nonetheless impacting health. Advanced techniques, such as infrared imaging and moisture mapping, offer powerful tools for detecting mold in walls, ceilings, and other concealed areas. Once identified, the removal and remediation of mold become paramount. This process must be thorough and often requires the expertise of professionals trained in the safe elimination of mold from indoor environments.

Addressing mold toxicity also involves a comprehensive look at one's lifestyle and daily habits. Simple changes, such as improving indoor air quality through the use of HEPA filters and ensuring adequate ventilation, can significantly reduce mold spore concentration in the air. Additionally, controlling humidity levels within the home is crucial, as mold thrives in moist environments. Dehumidifiers and air conditioners become valuable allies in maintaining a dry and mold-resistant living space.

Dietary adjustments play a pivotal role in mitigating the effects of mold exposure. A diet rich in anti-inflammatory foods and low in sugar can help bolster the body's defense against the inflammatory responses triggered by mycotoxins. Incorporating foods with natural antifungal properties, such as garlic, coconut oil, and ginger, can also support the body's ability to fight off mold-related health issues.

Supplementation is another critical component of the healing process. Specific vitamins, minerals, and antioxidants can aid in detoxifying the body from mycotoxins. For instance, glutathione, known as the body's master antioxidant, has been shown to support liver function and help in the elimination of toxins. Similarly, supplements like activated charcoal and bentonite clay can bind to mycotoxins in the gut, preventing their absorption and facilitating their removal from the body.

The psychological impact of living with mold toxicity and chronic illness is profound and often overlooked. It's essential to address the mental and emotional toll these conditions can take. Support groups, counseling, and therapies such as cognitive-behavioral therapy (CBT) can offer much-needed emotional support. Mindfulness practices, yoga, and meditation can also be beneficial in managing stress and improving mental well-being.

In conclusion, the journey to recovery from mold toxicity is multifaceted and requires a holistic approach that encompasses environmental, dietary, supplemental, and psychological strategies. By taking proactive steps to assess and remediate mold in their environments, individuals can significantly improve their health outcomes. Coupled with targeted nutritional and lifestyle interventions, it is possible to reduce the burden of mycotoxins and support the body's natural healing processes. As awareness grows and more resources become available, those affected by mold toxicity have a path forward toward regaining their health and vitality.

1.1: The Hidden Dangers of Mold Exposure

Mold's ability to proliferate in environments without overt signs is a significant health hazard, often going unnoticed until symptoms manifest. These microorganisms prefer damp, poorly ventilated areas, making basements, bathrooms, and kitchens prime locations for growth. However, they are not limited to these areas; mold can also be found behind walls, under carpets, and in ceiling tiles, areas not frequently inspected in daily life. The lack of visible indicators contributes to the silent spread of mold within living and working spaces, making it a stealthy adversary in the fight for health.

The toxins produced by mold, known as mycotoxins, are particularly insidious because they can become airborne and inhaled or attach to dust particles, making them easily ingested or inhaled without realization. Once inside the body, these toxins can disrupt normal cellular function, leading to a cascade of health issues. The symptoms associated with mold exposure are vast and varied, ranging from respiratory problems, such as coughing and wheezing, to more systemic issues like fatigue and neurological impairments. The broad spectrum of symptoms, coupled with their nonspecific nature, often leads to misdiagnosis or a dismissal of mold as a potential cause.

One of the most troubling aspects of mold exposure is its capacity to exacerbate existing health conditions. Individuals with asthma or immune disorders may find their symptoms worsening due to mold in their environment. Moreover, the presence of mold can trigger allergic reactions, which can range from mild to severe, further complicating the clinical picture. The challenge is compounded by the fact that reactions to mold are not universal; sensitivity varies greatly among individuals, making it difficult to establish a one-size-fits-all approach to diagnosis and treatment.

The detection of mold in one's environment is further complicated by the fact that mold can grow in places not easily visible or accessible. Traditional methods of mold detection, such as visual inspections, may not reveal the full extent of mold growth. This necessitates the use of more sophisticated techniques, such as air quality testing, which can detect the presence of mold spores in the air. However, these tests require specialized equipment and knowledge, making them less accessible to the average person.

The eradication of mold from an environment is no small feat. It requires identifying the source of moisture that allowed the mold to grow in the first place and addressing it to prevent future growth. Remediation efforts may range from simple cleaning with mold-killing solutions to extensive renovations to remove and replace mold-infested materials. The process can be costly and time-consuming, adding a layer of stress and financial burden to those already suffering from health issues related to mold exposure.

Preventative measures play a crucial role in combating mold growth. Simple actions, such as maintaining proper ventilation, using dehumidifiers in damp areas, and promptly addressing water leaks, can significantly reduce the risk of mold development. Regular cleaning and inspections of areas prone to mold growth can also help catch and address issues before they escalate into larger problems.

The hidden dangers of mold exposure underscore the importance of awareness and proactive measures in maintaining a healthy living environment. By understanding the conditions that favor mold growth and the potential health risks associated with exposure, individuals can take steps to protect themselves and their families from the insidious effects of mold. Through education, prevention, and prompt action when mold is detected, it is possible to mitigate the health impacts of this common yet often underestimated threat.

1.2: Mold's Impact on Body and Mind

Mold's influence extends beyond the physical, deeply affecting cognitive functions and emotional well-being. The toxins produced by mold, when inhaled or absorbed, can cross the blood-brain barrier, a protective shield designed to keep harmful substances away from the brain. Once these toxins bypass this barrier, they can cause a variety of neurological symptoms that significantly impact daily life. Individuals exposed to mold may experience memory loss, difficulty concentrating, and a phenomenon often referred to as "brain fog," where thinking becomes sluggish and unclear. These cognitive impairments can be particularly distressing, as they affect one's ability to perform at work, manage daily tasks, and maintain social relationships.

Moreover, the psychological ramifications of mold exposure are profound. The constant battle with chronic symptoms can lead to feelings of anxiety and depression. The uncertainty of a mold-related illness, coupled with the frequent misdiagnosis and lack of understanding from others, can exacerbate these feelings, creating a cycle of mental health challenges. It's not uncommon for individuals suffering from mold toxicity to feel isolated and misunderstood, further compounding their stress and emotional distress.

The impact on the nervous system can manifest in more direct physical symptoms as well. Some individuals report increased sensitivity to light and sound, headaches, and even episodes of vertigo or dizziness. These symptoms can be alarming and debilitating, making it difficult for those affected to engage in normal activities or feel safe in environments that were once comfortable.

Addressing these complex symptoms requires a holistic approach that considers both the physical and mental health aspects of mold exposure. Strategies to support cognitive function and emotional well-being are essential components of a comprehensive recovery plan. Nutritional interventions, such as incorporating foods rich in antioxidants and omega-3 fatty acids, can support brain health and reduce inflammation. Supplements like magnesium and B vitamins may also be beneficial in supporting neurological function and mitigating some of the cognitive effects of mold exposure.

For the emotional and psychological effects, counseling or therapy can be invaluable in providing support and coping strategies. Techniques such as cognitive-behavioral therapy (CBT) can help individuals reframe their experiences and develop healthier thought patterns. Mindfulness practices, including meditation and yoga, can offer additional tools for managing stress and anxiety, promoting a sense of calm and well-being.

It's also important for individuals dealing with mold toxicity to seek out supportive communities, whether online or in person. Connecting with others who have experienced similar challenges can provide a sense of understanding and camaraderie that is often missing in their immediate social circles. These connections can be a source of practical advice, emotional support, and encouragement on the journey to recovery.

In managing the cognitive and psychological effects of mold exposure, it's crucial to adopt a patient and compassionate approach. Recovery can be a slow process, with ups and downs along the way. Celebrating small victories and acknowledging progress, no matter how incremental, can help maintain motivation and a positive outlook. By addressing both the body and mind, individuals can work towards regaining their health, clarity, and vitality, moving beyond the shadows cast by mold toxicity.

1.3: Mold, Lyme Disease, and Chronic Illness Connection

The intricate relationship between mold exposure, Lyme disease, and various chronic illnesses is a complex puzzle that demands careful attention. Both mold toxicity and Lyme disease can trigger an array of similar symptoms, including but not limited to extreme fatigue, joint and muscle pain, cognitive impairment, and neurological issues. This symptom overlap often leads to confusion in diagnosis and, consequently, treatment. For individuals grappling with these health challenges, understanding this connection is pivotal in seeking appropriate care and interventions.

Lyme disease, caused by the Borrelia burgdorferi bacterium transmitted through tick bites, is notorious for its wide-ranging effects on the body, mirroring many of the symptoms induced by mold exposure. The situation is further complicated as mold toxicity can exacerbate the symptoms of Lyme disease, creating a vicious cycle of illness that can be challenging to break. This interplay between mold exposure and Lyme disease can significantly impact an individual's immune system, making it more difficult for the body to fight off infections and recover from illness.

The misdiagnosis issue arises when healthcare providers, unfamiliar with the nuanced effects of mold exposure, may attribute all symptoms to Lyme disease or another chronic condition, overlooking the critical role that mold toxicity plays in the patient's health. This oversight can lead to treatments that are at best incomplete and, at worst, ineffective, leaving patients struggling with ongoing health issues.

To navigate this complex health landscape, individuals suspecting mold exposure or Lyme disease should seek out medical professionals experienced in environmental medicine or those who specialize in complex chronic illnesses. These practitioners are more likely to consider a comprehensive range of diagnostic tests that can differentiate between mold toxicity, Lyme disease, and other chronic conditions. Key tests include specific markers for inflammation, immune response assessments, and tests for mycotoxins, alongside traditional Lyme disease testing methodologies.

For those living in environments where mold is present, or in areas endemic to ticks carrying Lyme disease, proactive measures can be a crucial part of maintaining health. Reducing exposure to mold through proper home ventilation, using dehumidifiers, and promptly addressing water leaks or dampness can mitigate mold growth. Similarly, protecting oneself from tick bites by using repellents, wearing protective clothing, and performing regular tick checks after spending time outdoors can reduce the risk of Lyme disease.

In cases where both mold exposure and Lyme disease are confirmed, a multi-faceted treatment approach that addresses both conditions is essential. This may include antibiotics or antimicrobial treatments for Lyme disease, alongside strategies to detoxify the body from mycotoxins, such as using binders and supporting liver function. Nutritional support, including a diet rich in anti-inflammatory foods and supplements to boost the immune system, can also play a vital role in recovery.

Moreover, addressing the environmental factors that contribute to mold exposure is critical. This may involve professional mold remediation, improving indoor air quality, and making lifestyle adjustments to minimize exposure to mold and other toxins. For individuals with Lyme disease, ongoing support to manage symptoms and prevent relapse is equally important, including physical therapy, pain management, and strategies to support mental and emotional well-being.

In conclusion, the intersection of mold exposure, Lyme disease, and chronic illness presents a challenging health dilemma that requires a nuanced understanding and approach to treatment. By recognizing the overlapping symptoms and potential for misdiagnosis, individuals can advocate for themselves and seek out specialized care that addresses the full spectrum of their health concerns. Through targeted interventions, environmental modifications, and supportive care, it is possible to navigate the complexities of these conditions and move toward recovery and improved quality of life.

1.4: Who This Book Is For

This book is an invaluable resource for adults grappling with unexplained health issues that have eluded diagnosis or effective treatment. It speaks directly to those who have been navigating the complexities of chronic illness, whether they are in the early stages of seeking answers or have been managing symptoms for an extended period without significant improvement. The content is meticulously designed to cater to a wide spectrum of readers, from those with a rudimentary understanding of mold toxicity and its implications to individuals well-versed in the subject but seeking deeper insights or new strategies for mitigation and healing.

For families striving to create a safe and healthy living environment, this guide offers practical advice on identifying potential hazards in the home and implementing measures to eradicate them. It underscores the importance of awareness and proactive management of indoor air quality to safeguard against the insidious health impacts of mold exposure.

Individuals managing chronic conditions such as Lyme disease, fibromyalgia, Chronic Inflammatory Response Syndrome (CIRS), and autoimmune disorders will find the discussions on the interplay between mold toxicity and these illnesses particularly enlightening. The book provides a comprehensive overview of the symptoms and mechanisms of mold-related health issues, empowering readers with the knowledge to advocate for appropriate medical testing and treatment options.

Moreover, the guide extends beyond the physical aspects of mold toxicity, acknowledging the psychological and emotional challenges that accompany chronic illness. It offers strategies for coping with the stress, anxiety, and isolation that often accompany these conditions, emphasizing the importance of mental and emotional well-being in the healing process.

In essence, this book serves as a beacon of hope and a practical manual for anyone affected by mold toxicity or chronic illness, providing the tools and knowledge necessary to navigate the path to recovery. It is a testament to the resilience of the human spirit and the possibility of reclaiming one's health and vitality through informed action and perseverance.

Chapter 2: Identifying Mold Toxicity

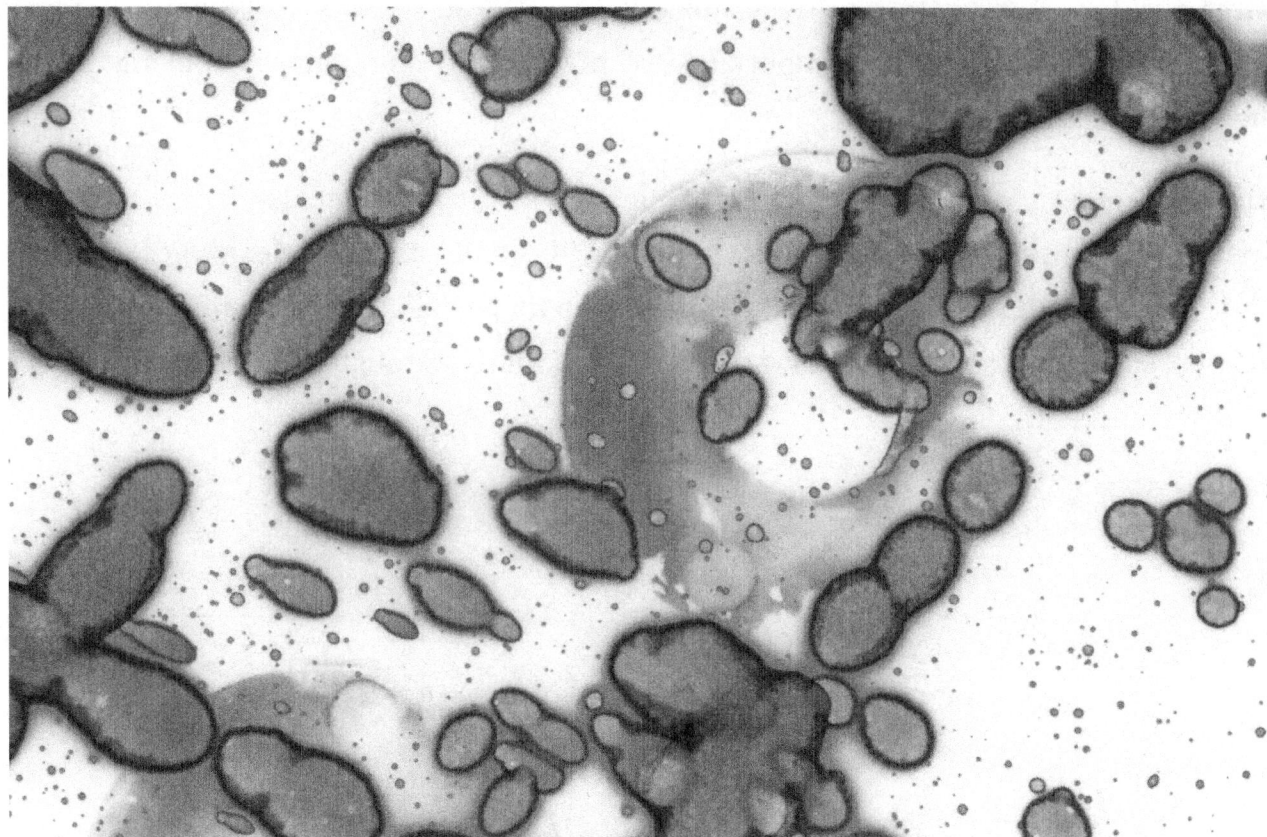

Identifying mold toxicity begins with recognizing the **common symptoms** associated with exposure to mold and its byproducts, mycotoxins. These symptoms can range widely, affecting various systems within the body, and may include chronic fatigue, headaches, sensitivity to light, respiratory issues, and cognitive disturbances such as difficulty concentrating or memory problems. It's crucial to understand that these symptoms can often mimic those of other conditions, making accurate identification challenging yet imperative for effective treatment.

The variability in symptoms is partly due to the **genetic predisposition** of individuals to mold sensitivity. Certain genetic markers can make some people more susceptible to the effects of mycotoxins, leading to a more pronounced response. This genetic aspect underscores the importance of personalized medical attention when addressing mold-related health issues.

Another critical step in identifying mold toxicity involves assessing one's **environment** for the presence of mold. Mold thrives in damp, poorly ventilated areas, and its detection is not always straightforward. Visible mold, musty odors, water damage, and excessive humidity are telltale signs, but mold can also reside in hidden areas, such as behind walls or under carpets. Therefore, a thorough inspection of one's living or working environment is essential, potentially requiring professional assistance for accurate assessment.

The **Mold Toxicity Self-Assessment Questionnaire** is a valuable tool for individuals suspecting they might be experiencing symptoms related to mold exposure. This comprehensive questionnaire covers a range of symptoms and exposure scenarios to help gauge the likelihood of mold toxicity. While not a substitute for professional medical diagnosis, this self-assessment can be a critical first step in identifying the need for further investigation and testing.

For those seeking a more definitive diagnosis, **medical testing** for mold exposure and sensitivity can provide concrete evidence of mold toxicity. Tests may include blood work to identify specific antibodies that react to mold, skin prick tests to determine allergic reactions, and urine tests for mycotoxin exposure. It's important to work with healthcare providers familiar with mold toxicity to ensure that the most appropriate and comprehensive tests are conducted.

Understanding the role of the environment in mold toxicity cannot be overstated. Indoor air quality tests can reveal the presence of mold spores and mycotoxins in one's surroundings, offering a clearer picture of exposure levels. These tests, while sometimes costly, can be instrumental in linking symptoms to mold exposure, especially in cases where physical symptoms are ambiguous or can be attributed to other causes.

In addressing mold toxicity, the **immediate reduction of exposure** is paramount. This may involve simple steps such as removing visible mold with safe cleaning solutions, using dehumidifiers to control indoor humidity, or more complex measures like professional mold remediation. The goal is to create a living environment that minimizes mold growth and exposure, thereby reducing the health risks associated with mold toxins.

Diet and lifestyle adjustments also play a critical role in managing symptoms of mold toxicity. A diet rich in anti-inflammatory foods and low in sugars can help mitigate the body's inflammatory response to mycotoxins. Additionally, certain supplements and herbs have been shown to support the body's detoxification processes, aiding in the elimination of toxins.

As we delve deeper into the strategies for detoxing the body from mold exposure, it's essential to consider the multifaceted approach required to address this complex health issue. From environmental modifications to dietary changes and medical interventions, each aspect of the detoxification and healing process is critical in restoring health and vitality in individuals affected by mold toxicity.

Environmental modifications are a cornerstone in the battle against mold toxicity. Ensuring that your living or working space is free from dampness and well-ventilated can drastically reduce mold growth. Regular inspections for leaks, proper installation of exhaust fans in high-moisture areas like bathrooms and kitchens, and the use of air purifiers equipped with HEPA filters can significantly improve indoor air quality. It's also beneficial to adopt habits that reduce indoor humidity, such as avoiding indoor line drying of clothes and ensuring that houseplants do not contribute to indoor moisture levels.

Professional mold remediation might be necessary in severe cases where mold infestation is extensive. This process typically involves isolating the contaminated area, removing affected materials, and employing air filtration devices to capture airborne spores. Post-remediation testing is crucial to ensure that the mold has been effectively removed. Selecting a reputable remediation service is vital, as improper remediation can spread mold throughout the home, exacerbating the problem.

On the dietary front, focusing on a nutrient-dense diet that supports the immune system and reduces inflammation is key. Foods rich in vitamins, minerals, and antioxidants can help the body resist and repair the damage caused by mycotoxins. Incorporating sources of healthy fats, lean proteins, and complex carbohydrates can provide the energy needed for recovery. Fermented foods and probiotics are beneficial for gut health, which is often compromised in individuals dealing with mold toxicity.

Supplementation can further aid in detoxification and recovery. Compounds such as N-acetylcysteine (NAC) support the production of glutathione, a critical antioxidant in the body's detoxification process. Omega-3 fatty acids, found in fish oil supplements, can help reduce inflammation, while milk thistle supports liver health, an essential organ in the detoxification process. It's important to consult with a healthcare provider before starting any new supplement regimen, especially for individuals with pre-existing health conditions or those taking other medications.

Hydration is another critical aspect of detoxification. Drinking adequate amounts of clean, filtered water helps to flush toxins from the body and supports all bodily functions. Engaging in regular, moderate exercise can also promote detoxification through sweating and improve overall well-being. However, it's crucial to listen to your body and not overexert, as individuals recovering from mold toxicity may have varying levels of physical tolerance.

The psychological aspect of dealing with mold toxicity should not be underestimated. The stress and anxiety that come with health issues can impede recovery. Practices such as mindfulness meditation, deep breathing exercises, and gentle yoga can help manage stress levels. Seeking support from therapists, counselors, or support groups familiar with environmental illnesses can provide emotional support and coping strategies.

Finally, ongoing vigilance is necessary to prevent re-exposure. This includes being mindful of environments outside of the home, such as workplaces or public buildings, that may also be sources of mold exposure. Educating oneself about the risks and maintaining a proactive stance on indoor air quality can help manage and mitigate the impacts of mold toxicity over the long term.

By adopting a comprehensive approach that includes environmental, dietary, and lifestyle changes, along with professional medical support, individuals can navigate the complexities of mold toxicity. With patience and persistence, it is possible to reduce exposure, detoxify the body, and support recovery, leading to improved health and a better quality of life.

2.1: Common Symptoms of Mold Exposure

Physical symptoms of mold exposure can range widely, reflecting the diverse ways in which individuals react to mycotoxins. Commonly reported physical symptoms include:

- **Respiratory problems**: Persistent coughing, wheezing, and shortness of breath are frequent signs. Individuals may also experience sinus congestion, nosebleeds, and sore throat.
- **Skin irritation**: Rashes, itching, and other skin irritations are common. Some individuals may develop hives or eczema in response to mold exposure.
- **Eye irritation**: Red, watery, itchy eyes are often reported, resembling allergic conjunctivitis.
- **Fatigue and weakness**: Unexplained chronic fatigue that does not improve with rest can be a significant indicator of mold-related illness.
- **Headaches and migraines**: Frequent headaches, including migraines that are resistant to typical treatments, can be linked to mold exposure.
- **Joint pain and muscle aches**: Unexplained muscle cramps, joint pain, and aches without clear cause or after physical activity.
- **Neurological symptoms**: Dizziness, memory loss, trouble concentrating, and confusion are neurological symptoms that some individuals experience.

Mental and emotional symptoms are equally important but can be more challenging to directly attribute to mold exposure due to their subjective nature. However, many individuals affected by mold toxicity report:

- **Cognitive difficulties**: Problems with focus, memory, and executive functions can be profound, often described as "brain fog."
- **Mood swings**: Individuals may experience rapid changes in mood, including irritability and anger, without a clear cause.
- **Anxiety and depression**: Increased levels of anxiety and episodes of depression can occur, which may be resistant to conventional treatments.
- **Sleep disturbances**: Difficulty falling asleep or staying asleep, leading to insomnia or non-restorative sleep, further exacerbating fatigue.

Emotional symptoms often stem from the chronic nature of mold-related illnesses and the frustration and isolation that can accompany them. These include:

- **Feeling overwhelmed**: The constant management of symptoms and the search for diagnosis and treatment can be overwhelming.
- **Social withdrawal**: Due to the chronic fatigue and other symptoms, individuals may withdraw from social activities they once enjoyed.
- **Frustration and hopelessness**: The difficulty in obtaining a clear diagnosis and effective treatment can lead to feelings of frustration and hopelessness.

It is crucial to recognize the variability in symptoms across individuals, as mold toxicity does not present uniformly. The wide range of symptoms, overlapping with other conditions, makes diagnosis and treatment challenging. Understanding this variability is key to recognizing and addressing mold-related illnesses effectively.

2.2: Chronic Illness or Mold Toxicity?

The challenge in distinguishing between symptoms of chronic illness and those caused by mold toxicity lies in their significant overlap. For instance, conditions such as **Chronic Fatigue Syndrome** (CFS) and **Fibromyalgia** share many symptoms with mold exposure, including profound fatigue, joint pain, and cognitive difficulties. This overlap not only complicates diagnosis but also can lead to mismanagement of the underlying condition if not accurately identified.

Lyme disease, another condition with symptoms that mimic those of mold toxicity, further complicates the diagnostic landscape. Both conditions can cause neurological issues, such as memory loss and difficulty concentrating, known colloquially as "brain fog." Additionally, the immune dysregulation seen in Lyme disease can be exacerbated by mold exposure, leading to a more severe presentation of symptoms.

The role of **genetic predispositions** cannot be overstated in this context. Certain individuals possess genetic markers, such as variations in the HLA-DR gene, that make them more susceptible to the effects of mycotoxins. This genetic vulnerability means that for some, exposure to mold can trigger a more severe or chronic response, closely mimicking or amplifying the symptoms of pre-existing conditions.

Understanding the **biological mechanisms** at play is crucial for accurate diagnosis and treatment. Mycotoxins can disrupt cellular processes and mitochondrial function, leading to widespread inflammation and oxidative stress. This biological disruption mirrors the pathophysiology of many chronic illnesses, making it difficult to discern the root cause of symptoms.

Diagnostic testing plays a pivotal role in differentiating between mold toxicity and other chronic conditions. Comprehensive blood panels, including markers of inflammation, immune response, and specific mycotoxin antibodies, can provide clues. Additionally, urine tests for mycotoxins offer direct evidence of mold exposure. However, it's important to note that these tests must be interpreted within the broader context of the patient's symptoms and medical history.

Environmental assessments are equally important. A thorough examination of the patient's living or working environment for mold can offer critical insights. Professional mold inspectors utilize tools such as moisture meters and infrared cameras to detect mold growth that may not be visible to the naked eye.

For individuals struggling with unexplained chronic symptoms, considering mold toxicity as a potential culprit is a crucial step. This requires a multidisciplinary approach, involving healthcare providers knowledgeable in both environmental medicine and the specifics of chronic illnesses. Treatment strategies often include **environmental remediation**, **detoxification protocols**, and **nutritional support** to address both the immediate effects of mold exposure and the underlying chronic condition.

In conclusion, the interplay between mold toxicity and chronic illness presents a complex diagnostic and therapeutic challenge. A detailed understanding of the symptoms, coupled with targeted testing and environmental assessment, is essential for untangling this intricate web. Through such an approach, individuals can embark on a path toward healing, addressing both the environmental and biological factors contributing to their condition.

2.3: Genetics and Mold Sensitivity

Genetic predispositions play a crucial role in determining an individual's sensitivity to mold and the severity of reactions they may experience upon exposure. The human leukocyte antigen (HLA) complex, a group of genes that regulate the immune system, has been identified as a significant factor in this sensitivity. Variations in the HLA gene can influence how an individual's body recognizes and responds to foreign substances, including mycotoxins produced by mold. Specifically, certain HLA-DR genotypes have been linked to a heightened susceptibility to chronic inflammatory response syndrome (CIRS), a condition associated with severe health effects from mold exposure.

Research indicates that individuals with these specific HLA-DR genotypes are unable to effectively recognize and eliminate mycotoxins from their bodies. This inability leads to an accumulation of toxins, triggering a chronic inflammatory response that can manifest in a wide array of symptoms, ranging from respiratory issues and cognitive impairments to chronic fatigue. It's estimated that approximately 24% of the population possesses these genetic variations, making them more vulnerable to mold-related health problems.

Moreover, the role of genetics does not stop with the HLA genes. Other genetic factors, including variations in detoxification pathways, can also influence an individual's sensitivity to mold. For instance, mutations in genes responsible for the production of glutathione S-transferases, enzymes crucial for detoxification, can impair the body's ability to process and eliminate mycotoxins. Similarly, mutations in the MTHFR gene, which plays a role in processing folate and regulating homocysteine levels, can impact the body's detoxification processes and immune function, further increasing susceptibility to mold toxicity.

Given the complexity of genetic influences on mold sensitivity, genetic testing can be a valuable tool for individuals experiencing unexplained health issues potentially related to mold exposure. Identifying specific genetic vulnerabilities can help tailor detoxification and treatment strategies to the individual's unique needs, enhancing the effectiveness of interventions aimed at mitigating mold toxicity. For example, individuals with identified detoxification pathway mutations may benefit from targeted nutritional support to boost their detoxification capacity, including supplements that enhance glutathione production or folate metabolism.

In addition to genetic testing, a comprehensive approach to addressing mold sensitivity should include environmental assessments to identify and mitigate mold exposure, alongside interventions to support detoxification and healing. Strategies such as improving indoor air quality, adopting a diet rich in nutrients that support detoxification, and utilizing supplements to aid in the elimination of mycotoxins can be particularly beneficial for those with genetic predispositions to mold sensitivity.

Ultimately, understanding the role of genetics in mold sensitivity underscores the importance of personalized approaches to diagnosis and treatment. By acknowledging the interplay between genetic factors and environmental exposures, individuals can adopt more effective strategies for managing their health in the face of mold toxicity.

2.4: Mold Toxicity Self-Assessment

The **Mold Toxicity Self-Assessment Questionnaire** is designed to help you evaluate whether your symptoms may be related to mold exposure. This tool is not a substitute for professional medical advice but can serve as a guide to understanding your health concerns better. Answer each question honestly and tally your responses to assess your potential risk.

1. **Have you experienced unexplained respiratory issues such as coughing, wheezing, or difficulty breathing in the past year?**
   - Yes
   - No

2. **Do you frequently suffer from sinus congestion, nosebleeds, or sore throats without a clear cause?**
   - Yes
   - No

3. **Have you noticed skin irritation, rashes, or eczema that cannot be explained by other known allergies or conditions?**
   - Yes
   - No

4. **Do you often have red, watery, or itchy eyes that feel similar to allergic reactions?**
   - Yes
   - No

5. **Are you experiencing chronic fatigue or weakness that doesn't improve with rest?**
   - Yes
   - No

Chapter 2: Identifying Mold Toxicity

6. Do headaches or migraines plague you more frequently than they used to, without a known trigger?
- Yes
- No

7. Have you dealt with unexplained joint pain or muscle aches that don't seem related to physical activity or known health issues?
- Yes
- No

8. Do you find yourself struggling with memory loss, trouble concentrating, or dizziness?
- Yes
- No

9. Have you noticed a significant change in your mood, such as increased irritability, anxiety, or episodes of depression?
- Yes
- No

10. Are sleep disturbances like insomnia or non-restorative sleep a regular part of your life now?
- Yes
- No

11. Do you feel overwhelmed by managing your health symptoms, leading to social withdrawal or feelings of isolation?
- Yes
- No

12. Have you lived in or frequently visited buildings where you have seen mold or water damage?
- Yes
- No

13. **Despite efforts to address your health concerns, do you feel your symptoms have been persistently misunderstood or misdiagnosed by healthcare providers?**
   - Yes
   - No

Scoring:
- **0-4 Yes Responses**: Your symptoms may not be directly related to mold exposure, but it's important to continue exploring other potential causes with your healthcare provider.
- **5-8 Yes Responses**: There is a moderate likelihood that your symptoms could be related to mold exposure. Consider consulting with a specialist in environmental medicine or a healthcare provider knowledgeable about mold toxicity.
- **9-13 Yes Responses**: Your symptoms strongly suggest that mold exposure could be a significant factor. Professional evaluation and testing for mold toxicity, as well as an environmental assessment of your home or workplace, are highly recommended.

This questionnaire aims to highlight the potential link between your symptoms and mold exposure, encouraging further investigation and professional consultation. Remember, each individual's situation is unique, and comprehensive testing and personalized treatment are crucial steps toward recovery.

Chapter 3: The Science of Mold Toxicity

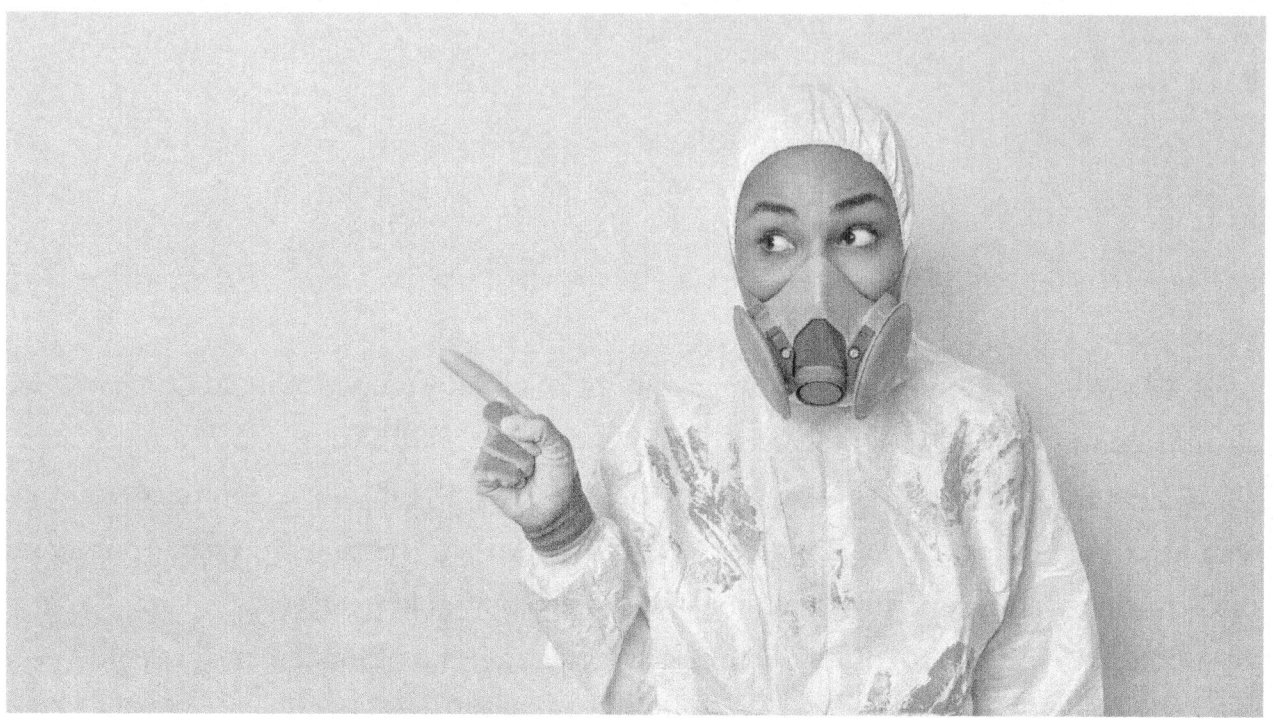

3.1: What Is Mold and Where It Thrives

Mold, a type of fungus, plays a crucial role in nature by breaking down dead organic matter. However, when it finds its way into our homes, it can become a significant health hazard. Mold thrives in moist, warm environments, often proliferating in places with poor ventilation or water damage. Understanding the various environments where mold can flourish is essential for preventing its growth and mitigating its impact on health.

Indoor Environments: Mold spores can enter homes through open doorways, windows, vents, and heating and air conditioning systems. Spores can also attach to clothing, shoes, and pets and be carried indoors. Inside, mold will grow in places with a lot of moisture, such as around leaks in roofs, windows, or pipes, or where there has been flooding. Common indoor habitats include damp basements, kitchens, bathrooms, and areas around heating and plumbing pipes.

Outdoor Environments: Outside, mold lives in soil, compost piles, and decaying leaves. It thrives in damp, shady areas and can proliferate on wood, paper, fabric, and other organic materials when moisture is present. While outdoor mold is less of a concern for direct health impacts than indoor mold, it can enter homes and buildings, increasing the indoor spore count.

High-Risk Environments: Certain environments are particularly susceptible to mold growth. These include:
- **Homes with poor ventilation**: Limited airflow encourages moisture buildup, creating an ideal environment for mold.
- **Buildings with water damage**: Flooding or leaks that are not promptly addressed can lead to extensive mold growth.
- **Humid climates**: Areas with high humidity levels can struggle with mold, as the air itself provides enough moisture for mold to thrive.
- **Construction materials**: Some building materials, like drywall, can absorb moisture and become breeding grounds for mold if exposed to water.

To prevent mold growth, it is crucial to control moisture levels in your home. This can be achieved by using dehumidifiers and air conditioners, especially in hot, humid climates, ensuring adequate ventilation in bathrooms, kitchens, and laundry areas, and addressing any leaks or water damage promptly. Additionally, using mold-resistant products in home construction and renovation can help prevent mold growth in high-risk areas.

Regular cleaning and maintenance of areas prone to moisture can also prevent mold from taking hold. For instance, cleaning gutters to prevent water buildup, ensuring the ground slopes away from your home's foundation to prevent water from collecting, and ventilating shower, laundry, and cooking areas can significantly reduce the risk of mold growth.

In summary, mold can thrive in various environments, particularly those with excessive moisture, poor ventilation, and organic materials to feed on. By understanding where mold is most likely to grow, individuals can take proactive steps to mitigate these risks, creating healthier living and working environments.

3.2: Mycotoxins and Their Health Impact

Mycotoxins, the toxic chemicals produced by mold, are a significant concern due to their ability to cause a wide range of health issues. These compounds are secondary metabolites of mold and can be found in various environments, particularly in areas with excessive moisture and decay. Understanding the nature of mycotoxins and their impact on the body is crucial for addressing mold toxicity effectively.

Mycotoxins can infiltrate the human body through inhalation, ingestion, or direct skin contact. Once inside, they can disrupt normal cellular processes, leading to a cascade of inflammatory responses. The liver, being the primary organ responsible for detoxification, bears the brunt of the effort to eliminate these toxins. However, the efficiency of the liver's detoxification pathways can vary significantly among individuals, influenced by genetic factors and overall health. This variability can lead to differences in susceptibility and response to mycotoxin exposure.

The **health impacts** of mycotoxins are vast and can manifest in numerous ways, depending on the type of mycotoxin, the level of exposure, and the individual's health status and genetic predisposition. Some of the most common health effects include:

- **Neurotoxic effects**: Certain mycotoxins can cross the blood-brain barrier, leading to neurological symptoms such as headaches, dizziness, and cognitive impairments.
- **Immunosuppression**: Prolonged exposure to mycotoxins can weaken the immune system, making the body more susceptible to infections and other diseases.
- **Hormonal disruption**: Mycotoxins can interfere with hormone production and regulation, potentially leading to endocrine disorders.
- **Respiratory issues**: Inhalation of mycotoxins can cause respiratory symptoms, including asthma, wheezing, and difficulty breathing.
- **Gastrointestinal problems**: Ingestion of mycotoxins can irritate the gastrointestinal tract, resulting in symptoms like nausea, vomiting, and diarrhea.

The **long-term impact** of mycotoxin exposure can be profound, with some studies suggesting a link between chronic exposure and the development of certain cancers, autoimmune diseases, and neurodegenerative conditions. The persistent inflammatory response triggered by mycotoxins can also contribute to the development of chronic inflammatory response syndrome (CIRS), a complex condition characterized by widespread inflammation and multiple system symptoms.

Given the serious health risks associated with mycotoxins, it is imperative to adopt strategies to minimize exposure and enhance the body's ability to detoxify these harmful compounds. Some recommendations include:

- **Improving indoor air quality**: Use HEPA filters in air conditioning and heating systems to reduce airborne mycotoxins.
- **Dietary adjustments**: Incorporate foods that support liver health and detoxification, such as leafy greens, cruciferous vegetables, and foods high in antioxidants.
- **Supplementation**: Certain supplements, including glutathione, milk thistle, and activated charcoal, can support detoxification pathways.
- **Environmental remediation**: Address mold growth in living and working environments promptly to reduce mycotoxin production.

In conclusion, mycotoxins represent a significant health hazard, particularly in environments with mold growth. By understanding the routes of exposure and the potential health effects, individuals can take proactive steps to reduce their risk and support their body's detoxification processes.

3.3: The Cell Danger Response

The cell danger response (CDR) is a fundamental survival mechanism that our bodies initiate in response to threats, including exposure to toxic substances like mycotoxins produced by mold. When the body detects these harmful agents, it triggers a protective cascade designed to mitigate damage. This response involves a complex network of signals that alter cellular function, metabolism, and immune system activity. However, when the exposure to mold is prolonged or the elimination of mycotoxins is not efficiently achieved, this once protective mechanism can become maladaptive, keeping the body in a perpetual state of alert. This persistent activation of the CDR can lead to a variety of chronic symptoms and illnesses, as the body's resources are continuously diverted towards survival rather than healing and regeneration.

Mycotoxins are particularly insidious in their ability to disrupt cellular function. They can bind to DNA, RNA, and proteins, leading to cellular damage and apoptosis. Furthermore, these toxins can impair mitochondrial function, which is crucial for energy production, leading to fatigue, one of the most common complaints among those affected by mold toxicity. The immune system is also heavily impacted, as the CDR promotes a shift towards a Th2-dominant response, which can exacerbate allergic reactions and reduce the body's ability to fight off infections.

One of the key challenges in overcoming the CDR is the body's reduced capacity to detoxify effectively. The liver, which plays a central role in the detoxification process, can become overwhelmed by the constant need to filter out mycotoxins. This can lead to a buildup of toxins in the body, further perpetuating the cell danger response. Additionally, the gut microbiome can be disrupted by mold exposure, impairing digestion and nutrient absorption, which are critical for detoxification and healing.

To support the body in moving out of survival mode and into a state conducive to healing, several strategies can be employed:

1. **Enhancing Detoxification**: Supporting liver function through dietary changes, supplements like milk thistle, and practices such as dry brushing and Epsom salt baths can help improve the body's ability to eliminate toxins. Incorporating foods rich in antioxidants and anti-inflammatory compounds can also support cellular repair and mitigate the effects of oxidative stress.

2. **Restoring Gut Health**: A healthy gut microbiome is essential for effective detoxification and immune function. Probiotics, prebiotics, and a diet rich in fiber can help rebuild a healthy gut flora. Eliminating foods that contribute to inflammation and gut dysbiosis, such as sugar and processed foods, is also crucial.

3. **Balancing the Immune Response**: Supplements like omega-3 fatty acids, vitamin D, and adaptogenic herbs can help modulate the immune system, reducing the Th2 dominance and promoting a more balanced immune response.

4. **Supporting Mitochondrial Function**: Nutrients like CoQ10, L-carnitine, and magnesium can support mitochondrial health, improving energy production and reducing fatigue.

5. **Mind-Body Practices**: Techniques such as meditation, yoga, and deep breathing exercises can help reduce stress and inflammation, promoting a shift away from the cell danger response.

By addressing the cell danger response directly and supporting the body's natural detoxification and healing processes, individuals suffering from mold toxicity can begin to recover and restore their vitality. It's important to approach recovery as a comprehensive process, addressing not just the physical symptoms but also the environmental and emotional factors that contribute to the condition.

Part 2:
Diagnosing Mold Exposure

Chapter 4: Medical Testing for Mold Illnesses

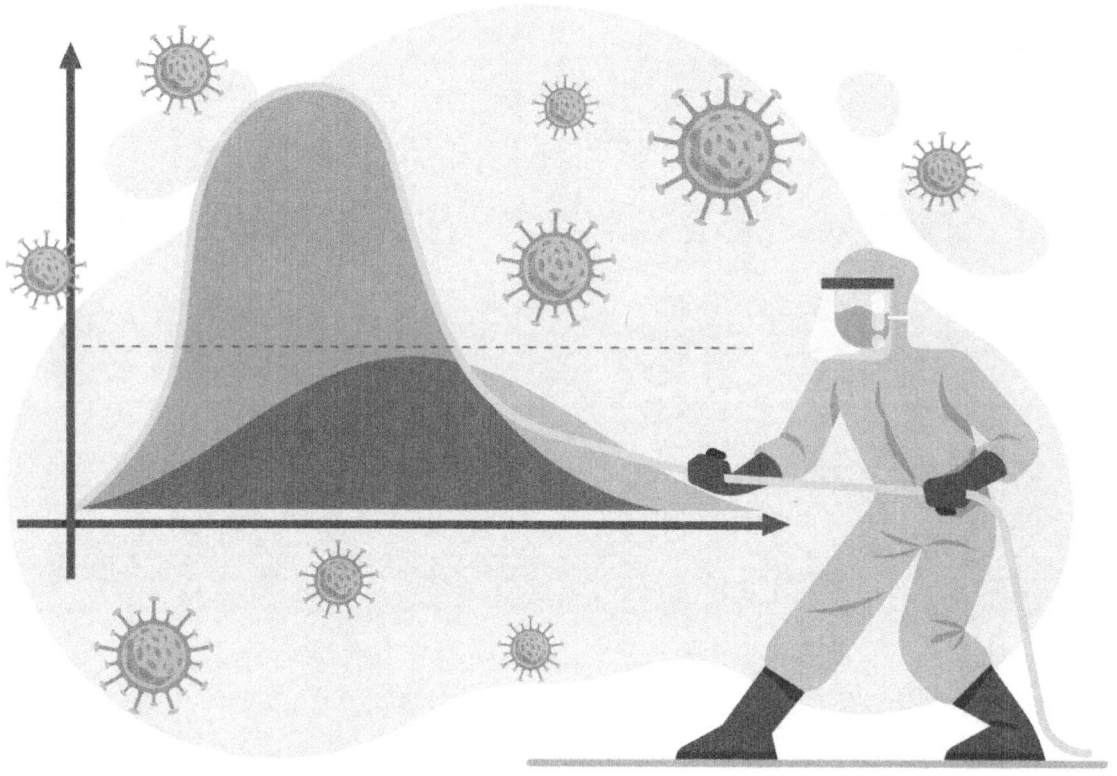

4.1: Key Medical Tests for Mold Toxicity

Upon suspecting mold toxicity, a series of **medical tests** can be instrumental in confirming the diagnosis. These tests are designed to detect the presence of mycotoxins in the body and assess the extent of the immune system's response to mold exposure. Understanding the specific tests and what they measure is crucial for individuals navigating the complexities of mold-related illnesses.

Blood Tests: Blood tests are often the first step in diagnosing mold toxicity. They can measure various markers indicative of an immune response to mold, including specific antibodies against mold species or mycotoxins. **C4a** is a marker of inflammation that can be elevated in cases of mold exposure. Additionally, tests for **HLA-DR** genotypes can identify individuals genetically predisposed to mold sensitivity, providing insight into why some people may suffer more severe reactions than others.

Urine Tests: Urine mycotoxin tests can directly measure the levels of mycotoxins excreted from the body. These tests are particularly valuable as they can identify specific mycotoxins, offering a clearer picture of the toxins involved. However, it's important to note that the presence of mycotoxins in urine does not necessarily confirm current mold exposure, as mycotoxins can remain in the body long after the initial exposure.

Visual Contrast Sensitivity (VCS) Test: While not a direct measure of mold toxicity, the VCS test can indicate the presence of neurotoxins, which are often produced by toxic mold. This simple and non-invasive test measures the ability to detect visual patterns of varying contrast and can be an early indicator of neurotoxin exposure.

Nasal Swab Test: For individuals experiencing chronic sinus issues, a nasal swab test can identify the presence of mold in the nasal passages. This test can be particularly revealing for those with persistent sinusitis, as mold colonization in the sinuses can be a significant source of ongoing mycotoxin exposure.

Comprehensive Diagnostic Approach: It's essential to approach the diagnosis of mold toxicity with a comprehensive strategy, utilizing a combination of these tests. No single test can confirm mold toxicity definitively, but together, they can provide a clearer picture of the body's exposure and response to mold. Consulting with a healthcare provider experienced in mold-related illnesses is crucial to interpret test results accurately and develop an effective treatment plan.

Interpreting Test Results: Understanding test results can be challenging, as the presence of mycotoxins or an immune response to mold does not necessarily correlate with the severity of symptoms. Some individuals may have high levels of mycotoxins but experience mild symptoms, while others with lower toxin levels may suffer severe health effects. This variability underscores the importance of a personalized approach to treatment, considering both test results and clinical symptoms.

In summary, the key to diagnosing mold toxicity lies in a comprehensive evaluation that includes a detailed medical history, symptom assessment, and targeted diagnostic tests. By accurately identifying the presence and impact of mold exposure, individuals can take informed steps toward recovery, guided by a tailored treatment strategy that addresses both the detoxification of mycotoxins and the restoration of health.

4.2: Testing for Mycotoxins

Testing for mycotoxins is a critical step in diagnosing mold exposure and its impact on health. Mycotoxins, toxic compounds produced by certain types of mold, can cause a wide range of health issues, from mild allergic reactions to serious chronic conditions. Understanding the process, accuracy, and appropriate timing for these tests can empower individuals to take control of their health in the face of mold exposure.

Mycotoxin tests primarily analyze urine samples to detect the presence of these toxins. The rationale behind using urine is that it reflects substances the body is actively eliminating, providing a snapshot of the internal toxic burden. Some tests may also use blood, tissue, or sputum samples, but urine tests are the most common due to their non-invasive nature and the body's process of toxin excretion through the urinary tract.

The accuracy of mycotoxin testing can vary depending on several factors, including the type of test used, the specific mycotoxins being tested for, and the individual's metabolic rate and detoxification efficiency. It's important to select a testing method that is sensitive and specific to the mycotoxins of concern. High-quality tests can detect low levels of mycotoxins, providing valuable information even when exposure levels are minimal or the toxins are being efficiently excreted by the body.

When considering the timing for mycotoxin testing, it's crucial to account for the individual's exposure history and symptomatology. Testing is most appropriate when there is a reasonable suspicion of mold exposure based on environmental assessments or when individuals present with symptoms consistent with mycotoxin poisoning, such as chronic fatigue, cognitive difficulties, and unexplained allergic reactions. Early testing, soon after suspected exposure, can help identify the problem before more severe health issues arise. However, it's also worth noting that mycotoxins can remain in the body for extended periods, so testing can still be relevant and informative even months or years after the initial exposure.

Interpreting the results of mycotoxin tests requires expertise. Elevated levels of specific mycotoxins can indicate past or ongoing exposure to mold, but they do not necessarily correlate directly with the severity of symptoms or the prognosis. A comprehensive approach, considering both test results and clinical evaluation, is essential for developing an effective treatment plan. It may involve detoxification strategies, dietary modifications, and environmental interventions to reduce further exposure.

In some cases, follow-up testing is recommended to monitor the effectiveness of treatment interventions and the body's progress in eliminating mycotoxins. These subsequent tests can provide insight into the body's detoxification capacity and help adjust treatment strategies as needed.

In conclusion, mycotoxin testing is a valuable tool in the diagnosis and management of mold-related health issues. By understanding how these tests work, their accuracy, and the appropriate context for their use, individuals can make informed decisions about their health and recovery journey. Working with healthcare providers knowledgeable in environmental medicine and mold toxicity is crucial to accurately interpret test results and implement a holistic treatment approach.

4.3: Diagnosing Lyme and Co-Infections

Diagnosing Lyme Disease and its co-infections, such as Bartonella and Babesia, requires a nuanced understanding of the interplay between these infections and mold exposure. The diagnostic process is multifaceted, incorporating both direct and indirect testing methods to accurately identify these conditions. Given the overlapping symptoms with mold toxicity, healthcare providers must employ a comprehensive approach to ensure an accurate diagnosis.

Direct Testing Methods: These involve identifying the presence of the pathogen itself or its genetic material in the body. For Lyme Disease, the most common direct test is the Polymerase Chain Reaction (PCR) test, which detects the DNA of Borrelia burgdorferi, the bacterium responsible for Lyme Disease. Similarly, PCR tests can identify DNA from Bartonella and Babesia pathogens. Another direct method is culture testing, where blood or tissue samples are cultured in a lab to encourage the growth of the bacteria, although this method is less commonly used due to its complexity and the slow growth rate of these bacteria.

Indirect Testing Methods: These tests look for the body's immune response to the infection rather than the pathogen itself. The Enzyme-Linked Immunosorbent Assay (ELISA) test is often the first step, screening for antibodies against Borrelia burgdorferi. If the ELISA test results are positive or equivocal, the Western Blot test is performed as a confirmatory test to detect specific antibodies to several proteins of the bacterium. For Bartonella and Babesia, indirect fluorescence antibody (IFA) testing is commonly used to measure the immune response to these pathogens.

Interpreting Test Results: The interpretation of test results for Lyme Disease and its co-infections is complex. False negatives can occur, especially in the early stages of infection when the body has not yet produced a significant antibody response. Conversely, false positives can result from cross-reactivity with other bacteria. Clinical correlation, considering the patient's symptoms and exposure history, is crucial in making an accurate diagnosis.

Challenges in Diagnosis: One of the primary challenges in diagnosing Lyme Disease and co-infections is the significant overlap in symptoms with mold toxicity, including fatigue, cognitive impairment, and joint pain. This symptom overlap can lead to misdiagnosis or delayed diagnosis. Additionally, individuals with mold toxicity may have compromised immune systems, affecting the accuracy of serological tests.

Advanced Testing Options: For cases where standard testing methods are inconclusive, more advanced options may be considered. These include the C6 Lyme Peptide ELISA, which detects a specific peptide of Borrelia burgdorferi, and the Tick-Borne Disease Serochip (TBD Serochip), which offers a more comprehensive screening for multiple tick-borne pathogens simultaneously. Advanced imaging techniques, such as SPECT scans, can also provide evidence of Lyme-related neurological involvement, although these are not diagnostic tests per se.

Treatment Considerations: Upon confirming a diagnosis of Lyme Disease or co-infections, treatment should be tailored to the individual, taking into account the presence of mold toxicity. This may involve a combination of antibiotic therapy, antiparasitic medications, and supportive treatments to address symptoms and underlying immune dysfunction. Collaboration between specialists in Lyme Disease, mold toxicity, and other relevant fields is essential to develop an effective, holistic treatment plan.

In conclusion, diagnosing Lyme Disease and co-infections in the context of mold exposure requires a careful, comprehensive approach. By employing a combination of direct and indirect testing methods, considering the patient's complete clinical picture, and acknowledging the complexities introduced by mold toxicity, healthcare providers can enhance the accuracy of diagnosis and improve outcomes for affected individuals.

Chapter 5: Testing Your Environment

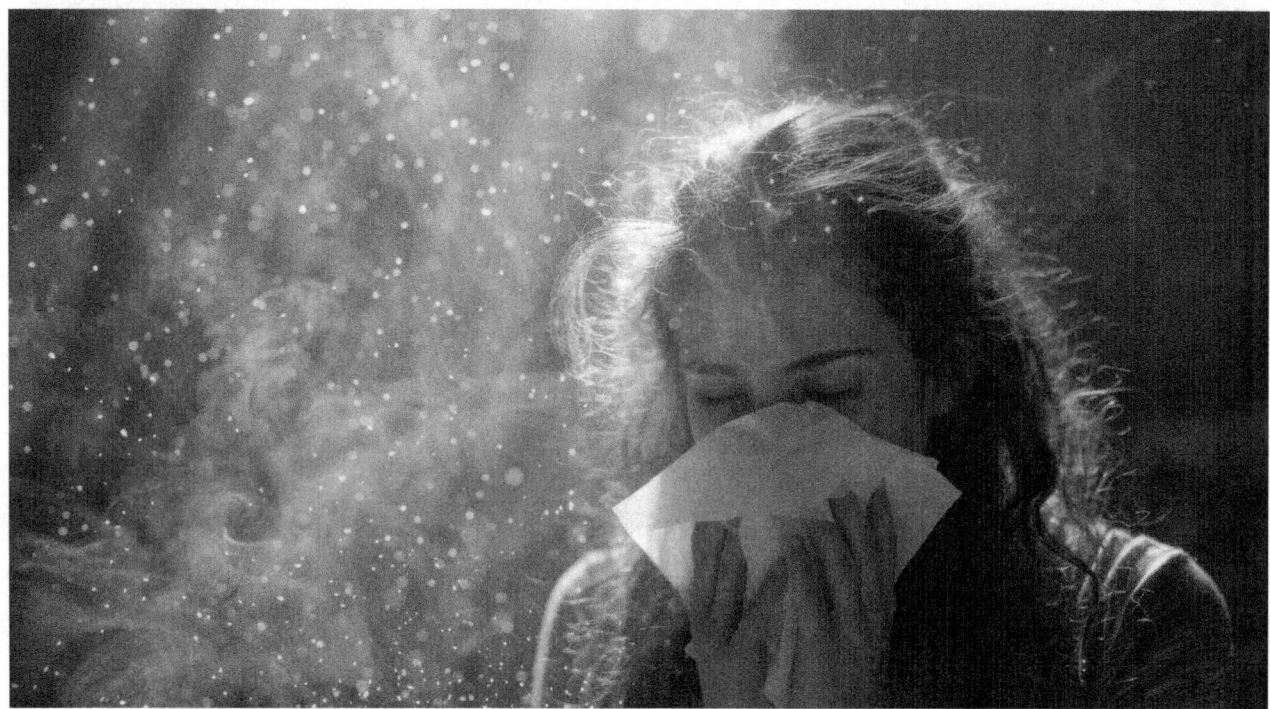

5.1: Detecting Mold in Your Home

After identifying the potential for mold growth through environmental assessments, the next crucial step is conducting a thorough visual inspection of your living spaces. This process involves meticulously examining areas where mold is most likely to proliferate, such as bathrooms, kitchens, basements, and around windows. Moisture is mold's best friend, so any signs of water damage, leaks, or condensation should be taken as red flags. Look for discoloration on walls, ceilings, and floors, which can range from black and green to white and orange spots, indicating different mold species. Peeling wallpaper or bubbling paint are also telltale signs that moisture has penetrated surfaces, creating a hospitable environment for mold.

In addition to visual cues, a musty odor is a strong indicator of hidden mold. This smell is distinctive and can help pinpoint areas where mold may be lurking out of sight, such as behind drywall or under carpets. Trust your nose; if an area smells damp or earthy, it's worth investigating further.

Moisture detection tools, such as hygrometers, can quantify the humidity levels in your home, providing concrete data to support your visual and olfactory findings. Ideal indoor humidity should be kept between 30% and 50% to discourage mold growth. Moisture meters, another valuable tool, can measure the moisture content of various materials, including wood, drywall, and carpeting. These instruments are particularly useful for detecting wet areas that are not visibly apparent.

For areas that are difficult to assess through visual inspection or with basic tools, consider employing thermal imaging technology. Infrared cameras can visualize temperature differences in walls and ceilings, revealing hidden moisture problems that would otherwise go unnoticed. While this technology can be more costly, it's an investment in accurately diagnosing mold issues, especially in large homes or in cases where mold is suspected but not visible.

Remember, the goal of these initial steps is to identify potential mold hotspots effectively. Once these areas are pinpointed, you can move forward with more detailed testing or professional assessments to confirm mold presence and species, laying the groundwork for a comprehensive remediation plan. Taking action at the first sign of mold is crucial to maintaining a healthy living environment and preventing the spread of mold throughout your home.

5.2: Professional vs. DIY Mold Testing

When considering the approach to mold testing, individuals are faced with two primary options: professional testing services or do-it-yourself (DIY) mold testing kits. Each method comes with its own set of advantages and potential drawbacks, which are crucial to understand for making an informed decision that aligns with one's needs, budget, and the severity of the mold issue at hand.

Chapter 5: Testing Your Environment

Professional Testing Services offer comprehensive assessments conducted by experienced technicians. These experts utilize advanced equipment to detect mold spores, identify the species of mold present, and assess the extent of mold contamination. The major advantage of professional testing is the accuracy and depth of analysis, which can pinpoint hidden mold and air quality issues not visible to the naked eye. Additionally, professional testers can provide detailed reports and recommendations for remediation. However, the cost of these services can be significantly higher than DIY methods, potentially running into hundreds or even thousands of dollars depending on the size of the area being tested and the complexity of the mold issue.

On the other hand, **DIY Mold Testing Kits** are readily available at home improvement stores and online, offering a more affordable option for initial mold detection. These kits typically include petri dishes or tape lifts that collect mold spores from the air or surfaces. After a specified period, the samples are sent to a lab for analysis, with reports sent back to the consumer. The benefits of DIY testing include lower upfront costs and the convenience of conducting the test at one's own pace. However, the limitations of these kits cannot be overlooked. They may not provide as comprehensive a picture as professional testing, potentially missing mold that is hidden or not airborne. Furthermore, the accuracy of DIY tests can vary, and interpreting the results without expert knowledge can be challenging.

When weighing **Professional Testing vs. DIY Testing**, consider the following factors:

- **Severity of Mold Issue**: For extensive or hidden mold problems, professional testing is more thorough.
- **Cost Consideration**: If budget constraints exist, a DIY kit may be a starting point, but understand its limitations.
- **Accuracy and Reliability**: Professional services offer detailed insights and accuracy.
- **Post-Testing Support**: Professionals can guide the next steps and remediation, unlike DIY kits.

Ultimately, the choice between professional mold testing and DIY kits depends on individual circumstances, including the urgency of the situation, the area's size suspected of mold growth, and budget constraints. For those experiencing severe health symptoms or suspecting widespread mold, investing in professional testing may yield a more accurate diagnosis and effective remediation plan. Conversely, for individuals simply seeking a preliminary assessment or who have visible mold in a small, contained area, a DIY mold testing kit might provide a cost-effective initial screening. Regardless of the chosen method, addressing mold issues promptly and effectively is crucial to maintaining a healthy living environment.

5.3: Interpreting Test Results

Once you have the results from either professional testing services or a DIY mold testing kit, the next crucial step is interpreting these findings to determine the safety of your environment and whether remediation is necessary. The complexity of test results can vary, but understanding the key indicators of mold presence and the potential health risks they pose is essential for making informed decisions about your next steps.

Mold Spore Count and Types: Test results often include a count of mold spores found in the sample and may identify specific types of mold present. High spore counts or the presence of certain mold types known for producing mycotoxins, such as Stachybotrys (commonly known as black mold), can indicate a significant health risk, necessitating professional remediation.

Comparison to Outdoor Levels: Many reports will compare indoor mold spore levels to those found outdoors. Indoor levels significantly higher than outdoor levels suggest that mold is growing and proliferating inside your home, which is a clear sign that action is needed to address the source of mold growth.

Mycotoxin Presence: If your testing included analysis for mycotoxins, the presence of these toxic compounds produced by mold can indicate a serious health risk. Mycotoxins can persist even after mold itself has been removed, so their detection may require more extensive cleaning and detoxification of your home environment.

Moisture Levels: Results that include information on moisture levels in your home can also guide your remediation efforts. High moisture levels can encourage mold growth, so addressing leaks, improving ventilation, and controlling humidity may be necessary steps alongside mold removal.

Interpreting Visual and Olfactory Evidence: In addition to laboratory results, do not discount visual signs of mold growth or musty odors as these can indicate problem areas not captured by testing. Sometimes, the most significant issues are hidden behind walls or under floors, so a professional evaluation might be necessary if these signs are present despite inconclusive test results.

Professional Consultation: For complex situations or when health symptoms persist, consulting with a mold remediation specialist or an environmental health professional can provide clarity. These experts can offer a more nuanced interpretation of test results, considering the unique aspects of your home and health situation.

Deciding on Remediation: If test results confirm mold presence at levels that pose health risks, or if there are visible signs of mold growth, professional remediation is often the safest course of action. Remediation should address not only the removal of mold but also the underlying moisture issues to prevent recurrence.

DIY Remediation Considerations: For minor mold issues confined to small areas (less than 10 square feet), DIY remediation may be feasible. This includes cleaning hard surfaces with detergent and water, ensuring the area is thoroughly dried, and possibly using HEPA vacuuming. However, protective gear and strict safety measures should be observed to prevent exposure to mold and mycotoxins.

Post-Remediation Testing: After remediation, conducting another round of testing can verify that mold levels have been reduced to safe levels and that the remediation efforts were successful. This step is crucial for ensuring the health and safety of your home environment.

Understanding your test results is the foundation for taking appropriate action to ensure your home is safe and healthy. Whether you opt for professional remediation or tackle minor issues yourself, the goal is to address both the mold and its underlying causes to create a safer, mold-free living space.

Part 3:
Protocols to Detox and Heal

Chapter 6: Creating a Mold-Free Environment

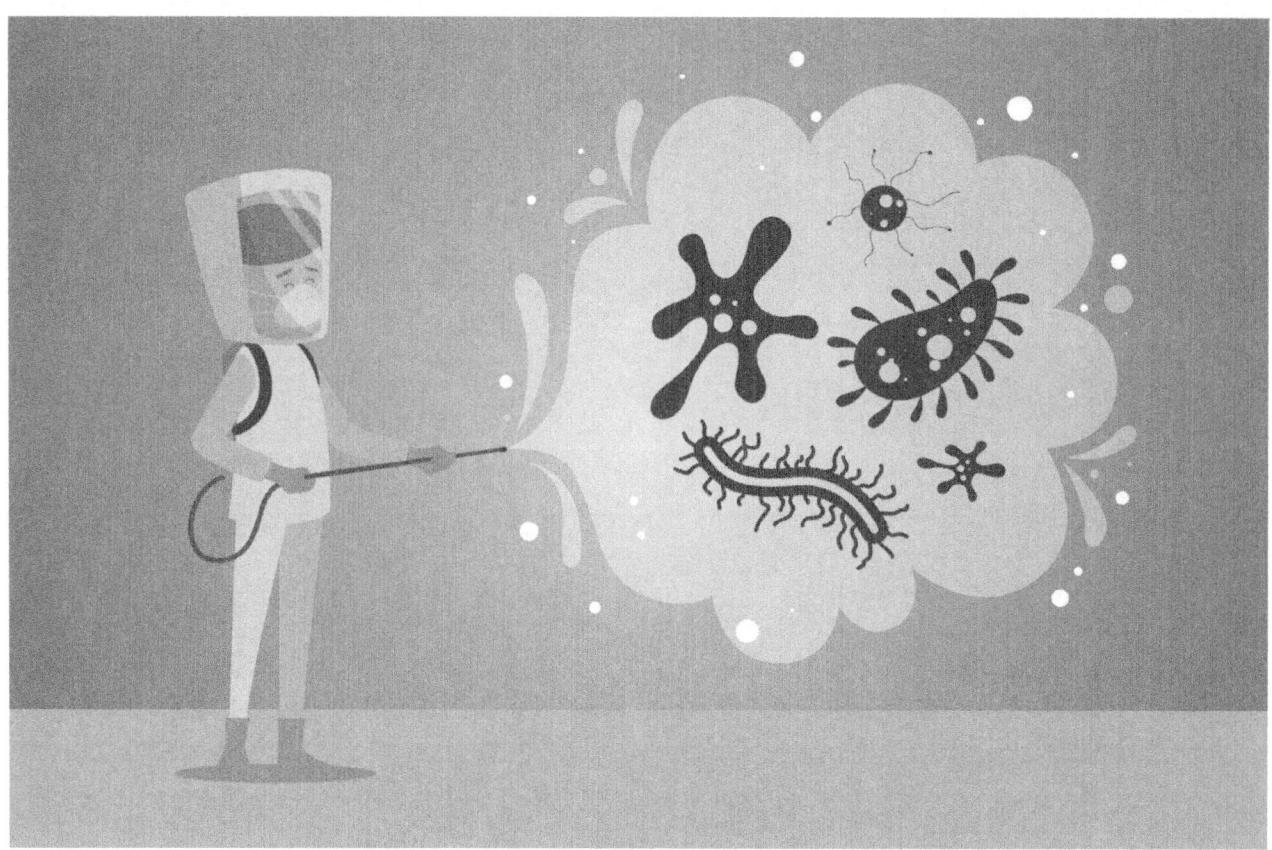

6.1: Immediate Steps to Reduce Mold Exposure

In the critical period before professional remediation can begin, taking immediate steps to reduce your exposure to mold is paramount. Here are actionable measures you can implement right away to safeguard your health and minimize further contamination:

1. **Isolate Affected Areas**: Close off any rooms or sections of your home where mold is visibly present or suspected. Use plastic sheeting and tape to seal doors and vents, preventing spores from spreading to other parts of your dwelling.

2. **Enhance Ventilation**: Increase airflow in your home by opening windows and using fans, but only in areas not affected by mold. This helps reduce moisture levels, a key factor in mold growth. However, avoid using fans if mold is present in the room, as this can spread spores.

3. **Use Air Purifiers**: Equip your home with HEPA air purifiers, especially in bedrooms and living areas. These devices can capture mold spores from the air, reducing your inhalation of these harmful particles.

4. **Address Moisture Sources**: Identify and rectify any sources of moisture, such as leaks in roofs, walls, or plumbing. Use dehumidifiers in damp areas like basements and bathrooms to keep humidity levels below 50%.

5. **Discard Contaminated Items**: Soft, porous materials like carpets, upholstered furniture, and curtains that have mold growth should be disposed of properly. Seal them in plastic bags to prevent spores from escaping during removal.

6. **Clean Non-Porous Surfaces**: Surfaces such as metal, glass, and plastic can be cleaned with a mixture of water and detergent. Avoid using bleach, as it does not prevent mold from returning and can pose health risks when mixed with mold spores.

7. **Protect Yourself During Cleaning**: Wear protective gear, including gloves, N95 masks, and goggles, to avoid direct exposure to mold and cleaning agents. Ensure good ventilation if you must clean areas with mild mold contamination.

8. **Limit Use of HVAC Systems**: If mold is suspected in ductwork or near HVAC units, limit the use of heating and cooling systems until they can be inspected. This prevents the spread of mold spores throughout your home.

9. **Inspect for Hidden Mold**: Check less visible areas where mold might grow, such as under sinks, behind appliances, and inside wall cavities. If you discover mold in these places, professional assessment is necessary.

10. **Stay Informed About Mold**: Educate yourself and your family about the risks of mold exposure and the importance of prompt action to address any signs of growth. Knowledge is a powerful tool in preventing mold-related health issues.

By implementing these steps, you can significantly reduce your exposure to mold and protect your health while waiting for professional remediation. Remember, these measures are temporary solutions. Comprehensive mold removal and addressing the underlying moisture issues are essential for a long-term resolution.

6.2: DIY Mold Remediation Guide

When embarking on DIY mold remediation, it's crucial to understand the scope of what you can safely handle and when it's imperative to call in professionals. The primary goal is to eradicate mold effectively while ensuring your safety and preventing further contamination. Here are detailed steps and precautions for tackling mold issues on your own, along with clear indicators that professional intervention is necessary.

Safety First: Before you begin, equip yourself with personal protective gear. This includes wearing an N95 respirator mask, gloves, goggles, and clothing that covers your entire body, which should be washed immediately after your remediation work. Ensuring proper ventilation in the area you're working in is also crucial; however, avoid using fans if they spread mold spores to other areas.

Identify the Mold Source: Start by identifying the moisture source that's contributing to mold growth. This could be a leaky pipe, condensation, or inadequate ventilation. Addressing this issue is critical to prevent mold from returning after you've cleaned it up.

Isolate the Contaminated Area: Seal off the area where mold is present to prevent spores from spreading to other parts of your home. Use plastic sheeting and tape to cover doorways, vents, and other openings.

Cleaning Small Areas: If the mold covers an area less than 10 square feet, it's generally considered safe to clean it yourself. Use a detergent solution to scrub mold off hard surfaces and then dry the area thoroughly. For absorbent materials like carpet or ceiling tiles, if mold has penetrated deeply, these items should be discarded properly.

Avoid Bleach: Contrary to popular belief, bleach is not recommended for mold remediation. It can cause mold spores to become airborne and does not prevent mold from returning. Instead, use solutions designed specifically for mold cleanup.

Dry the Area Completely: Mold thrives in moist environments, so it's essential to dry out the affected area thoroughly after cleaning. Use dehumidifiers and fans to help reduce moisture. Keep in mind that fans should not be used if they spread mold spores to other areas.

Dispose of Moldy Materials: Materials that cannot be cleaned should be sealed in plastic bags before being removed from your home to prevent the spread of spores. This includes anything from drywall and insulation to carpeting and fabric.

When to Call Professionals: If the mold covers an area larger than 10 square feet, if there's significant water damage, or if HVAC systems are contaminated, it's time to call in certified mold remediation professionals. Other scenarios that require professional intervention include mold caused by sewage or other contaminated water and situations where mold returns after repeated cleaning. Professionals have the equipment, training, and protective gear to handle large-scale mold problems safely and effectively.

Post-Remediation Testing: After the cleanup, whether done by you or professionals, it's wise to have the air quality tested to ensure all mold spores have been removed. This step is crucial for confirming the effectiveness of the remediation process.

Prevent Future Growth: Finally, take proactive measures to prevent mold from returning. This includes maintaining low indoor humidity levels (ideally between 30-50%), promptly repairing any leaks, and ensuring good ventilation throughout your home.

By following these guidelines, you can tackle minor mold issues safely on your own. However, recognizing when the situation is beyond your capabilities and requires professional remediation is crucial to protecting your health and your home. Remember, effectively dealing with mold is not just about cleaning up what's visible; it's about creating an environment where mold can't thrive in the first place.

6.3: Hiring Mold Remediation Professionals

When you decide to hire professionals for mold remediation, it's crucial to ensure you're choosing a reputable company that will effectively address the mold issue without causing further problems. Here are some tips to guide you through the selection process and what to expect during the remediation:

1. **Research and Referrals**: Start by researching local mold remediation companies. Look for businesses with positive reviews and testimonials. Referrals from friends, family, or professionals like home inspectors or real estate agents can also be invaluable.

2. **Certifications and Insurance**: Verify that the company holds relevant certifications in mold remediation. Organizations such as the Institute of Inspection, Cleaning and Restoration Certification (IICRC) or the National Organization of Remediators and Mold Inspectors (NORMI) provide standards for the industry. Additionally, ensure the company is insured to protect against potential damages during the remediation process.

3. **Detailed Inspection and Assessment**: A reputable company will start with a thorough inspection of your property to assess the mold situation. Expect them to provide a detailed report outlining the extent of the mold growth, the types of mold present, and the proposed method of remediation. This assessment should also include moisture measurements to identify the source of water contributing to the mold issue.

4. **Written Estimates**: Obtain written estimates from multiple companies. These should be detailed, listing the steps of the proposed remediation process, the timeline, and the cost. Be wary of quotes that seem significantly lower than others; this could indicate a lack of thoroughness or hidden costs.

5. **Containment and Safety Measures**: The remediation process should include proper containment of the affected area to prevent the spread of mold spores to other parts of your home. Ask about the safety measures they will use to protect their workers

and your home, such as HEPA air filtration devices and personal protective equipment (PPE).

6. **Communication**: Effective communication is key. The company should be willing to answer your questions and explain the remediation process in detail. They should also inform you of any unexpected issues that arise during the project and how they plan to address them.

7. **Post-Remediation Report and Guarantee**: After the remediation, the company should provide a post-remediation report detailing the work completed and the results of post-remediation testing, if conducted. Look for companies that offer a guarantee on their work, ensuring that if mold returns within a certain period, they will address it at no extra cost.

8. **Avoiding Scams**: Be cautious of companies that use scare tactics or claim to have a "secret method" for mold removal. Reliable remediation follows established protocols and standards. Also, be wary of companies that offer both testing and remediation services, as this can be a conflict of interest.

9. **Preparation for Remediation**: Before the company arrives, you may be asked to move furniture or belongings away from the affected area. Valuables and sensitive items should be secured. Depending on the extent of the remediation, you might also need to arrange for temporary accommodation for your family and pets to ensure safety and comfort.

10. **Follow-Up and Prevention**: After remediation, discuss with the company steps you can take to prevent mold from returning. This might include improving ventilation, fixing leaks, and controlling humidity levels in your home.

By following these guidelines, you can select a mold remediation company that will effectively and safely return your home to a healthy environment. Remember, the goal is not just to remove the mold but to address the underlying issues that allowed it to grow, ensuring your home remains safe and mold-free in the long term.

6.4: Preventing Mold Regrowth

Maintaining a mold-free environment requires a vigilant approach to **humidity control**, **ventilation**, and **regular inspections**. High humidity levels are a breeding ground for mold. It's essential to keep indoor humidity below 50% to prevent mold growth. This can be achieved through the use of dehumidifiers and air conditioners, especially during hot, humid months. Ensure that these appliances are cleaned and serviced regularly to function efficiently.

Ventilation plays a crucial role in preventing mold. Areas of your home that are prone to moisture, such as bathrooms, kitchens, and laundry rooms, should be well-ventilated. Exhaust fans that vent to the outside are particularly effective in these spaces. Opening windows and doors when weather permits also helps to reduce moisture and keep air circulating.

Regular inspections of your home can catch potential mold problems before they escalate. Pay special attention to places where water has the potential to accumulate, such as window sills, under sinks, and around appliances like refrigerators and dishwashers. Fix leaks promptly, no matter how small they may seem. Water damage can lead to mold growth in as little as 24-48 hours.

In addition to these strategies, consider the use of mold-resistant products when renovating or repairing your home. Mold-resistant drywall, paints, and building materials can provide an extra layer of protection against mold growth. For existing mold issues, cleaning with solutions designed to kill mold can be effective for small areas. However, for larger infestations, professional remediation may be necessary.

Moisture control is another critical aspect. Ensure that the ground around your home slopes away from the foundation to prevent water from collecting and seeping into the basement or crawl spaces. Gutters and downspouts should be clean and direct water away from your home. Additionally, inspect your roof regularly for damage that could allow water to enter your home.

By implementing these strategies, you can create a living environment that is less hospitable to mold. Remember, the key to preventing mold regrowth is to control moisture, improve air quality, and remain vigilant about home maintenance. Regularly cleaning and drying areas of your home that are susceptible to moisture, such as showers and sinks, can also prevent mold from taking hold.

Chapter 7: Detoxing Your Body

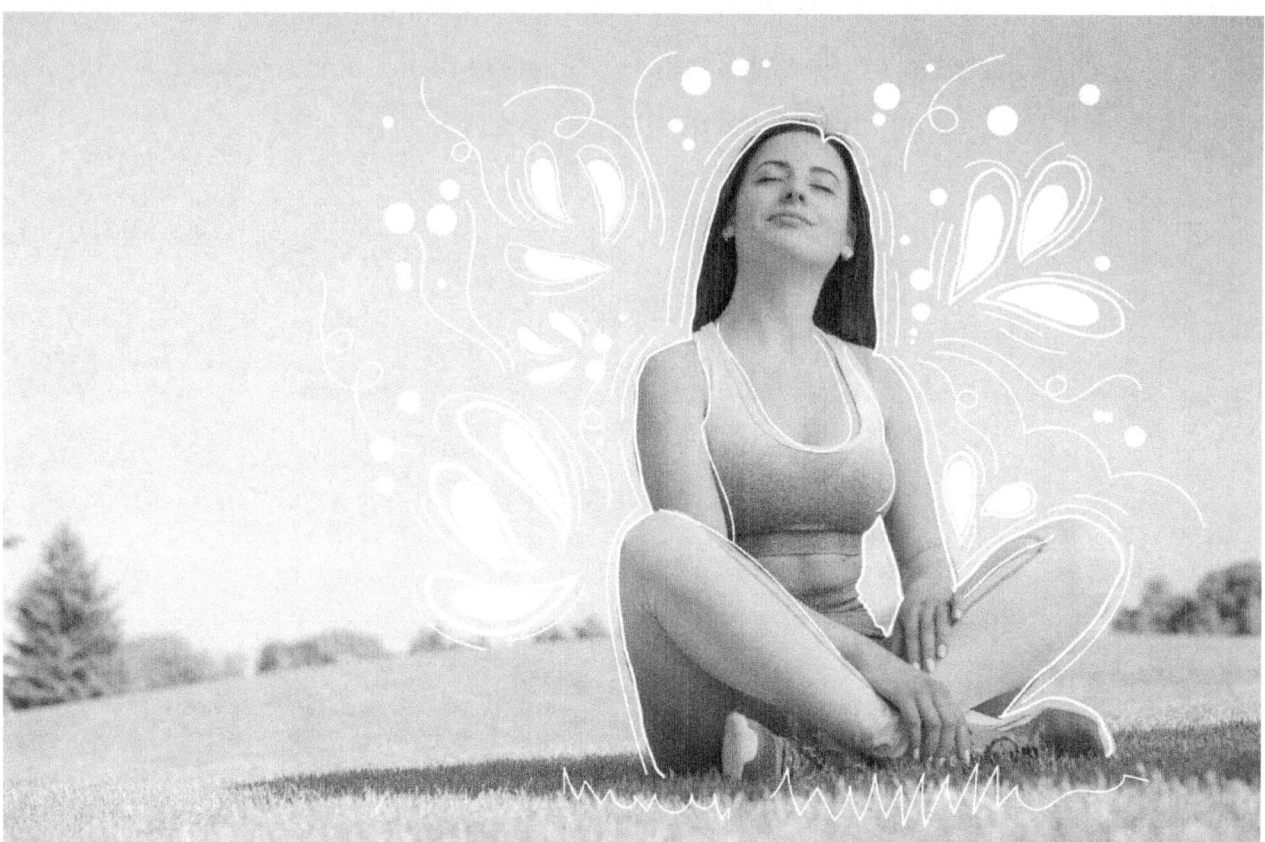

Detoxifying your body from mold exposure involves a multifaceted approach, focusing on supporting the liver, enhancing detox pathways, and incorporating nutritional strategies that bolster your body's natural ability to cleanse itself of toxins. The liver plays a pivotal role in detoxification, acting as the body's primary filtration system to neutralize and eliminate toxins. Enhancing liver function can be achieved through a diet rich in antioxidants and foods known for their liver-supporting properties. Foods such as leafy green vegetables, beets, garlic, and cruciferous vegetables like broccoli and Brussels sprouts are highly beneficial. These foods help increase the liver's detoxification enzymes, aiding in the more efficient processing of toxins.

In addition to dietary changes, certain supplements can provide targeted support for liver health and detoxification. Milk thistle, for example, is widely recognized for its liver-protective qualities. It contains silymarin, a compound that supports liver function by promoting the regeneration of liver cells and protecting against the entry of harmful toxins. Another valuable supplement is N-acetylcysteine (NAC), which boosts the production of glutathione, a critical antioxidant in the body's detoxification process. Glutathione plays a crucial role in neutralizing harmful free radicals and aiding in the metabolism of toxins.

Nutritional strategies extend beyond just supporting the liver. A diet that emphasizes anti-inflammatory foods can significantly impact your body's ability to detoxify from mold exposure. Incorporating a wide variety of colorful fruits and vegetables ensures a broad spectrum of vitamins, minerals, and antioxidants that combat inflammation and support overall health. Foods rich in fiber, such as legumes, whole grains, and seeds, are essential for maintaining a healthy gut microbiome, which is vital for proper detoxification and elimination of toxins.

Hydration is another key component of detoxification. Drinking adequate amounts of filtered water throughout the day helps to flush toxins from the body and supports kidney function. Herbal teas, such as dandelion or green tea, can be beneficial due to their diuretic properties and antioxidant content, further supporting the detox process.

Key supplements and herbs play a significant role in mold recovery by supporting detoxification pathways and providing antioxidant protection. Supplements like activated charcoal and bentonite clay can bind to toxins in the gut, preventing their absorption and facilitating their elimination from the body. However, it's important to use these supplements under the guidance of a healthcare professional, as they can also bind to essential nutrients and medications, potentially interfering with their efficacy.

Herbs such as cilantro and chlorella have been shown to have detoxifying properties, especially in the context of heavy metal and toxin removal from the body. Cilantro, in particular, is known for its ability to chelate, or bind to, heavy metals, making it easier for the body to eliminate them. Chlorella, a type of green algae, supports detoxification by binding to toxins and enhancing antioxidant status within the body. These natural detoxifiers can be incorporated into the diet or taken as supplements to aid in the body's cleansing processes.

The role of sauna and sweating in detox cannot be overstressed. Infrared saunas are a powerful tool for promoting detoxification through the skin, one of the body's primary elimination routes. The deep penetration of infrared heat raises the body's core temperature, stimulating sweat production and the release of stored toxins. Regular sessions can help reduce the body's toxin burden significantly. It's important to stay hydrated and replenish electrolytes when using saunas to support detoxification.

Exercise, while often overlooked, is another crucial element in the detoxification process. Engaging in regular physical activity increases blood flow and lymph circulation, enhancing the body's ability to expel toxins. Gentle exercises, such as walking, yoga, or swimming, can be particularly beneficial for those recovering from mold toxicity, as they stimulate detoxification without overburdening the body.

Managing stress and supporting the body's stress response are also vital components of a comprehensive detox plan. Chronic stress can impair the body's detoxification pathways, leading to increased toxin accumulation. Practices such as mindfulness meditation, deep breathing exercises, and yoga can help reduce stress levels, thereby supporting the body's natural detoxification processes.

Lastly, ensuring adequate sleep is paramount in supporting the body's healing and detoxification efforts. Sleep allows the body to repair and regenerate, processes that are critical for effective detoxification. Establishing a regular sleep schedule, creating a restful sleeping environment, and avoiding stimulants before bedtime can help improve sleep quality and, by extension, the body's ability to detoxify.

Incorporating these strategies into a holistic approach to detoxification can significantly enhance the body's ability to recover from mold exposure. It's essential to approach detox as a gradual process, allowing the body time to adjust and heal. With patience and consistency, these methods can support the body in clearing toxins, leading to improved health and vitality.

7.1: Supporting Liver and Detox Pathways

To further enhance the liver's detoxification capabilities, integrating specific lifestyle changes alongside dietary adjustments can significantly amplify the body's resilience against mold toxins. Regular physical activity, not only aids in toxin elimination through increased circulation and sweat but also boosts liver function by reducing fat deposits around the liver, a common impediment to its optimal performance. Aim for at least 30 minutes of moderate exercise daily, such as brisk walking or cycling, to maintain a healthy liver.

Stress management is another crucial aspect of supporting liver health and detox pathways. Chronic stress can lead to an accumulation of toxins in the body by hampering the liver's ability to filter blood efficiently. Techniques such as mindfulness meditation, deep breathing exercises, and yoga can help mitigate stress levels, thereby facilitating a more effective detox process.

Ensuring adequate sleep is paramount for liver health. The liver's detoxification processes are most active during the sleep cycle, particularly between 1 am and 3 am. Establishing a consistent sleep schedule that allows for 7-9 hours of quality sleep each night can significantly support the liver's natural detoxification rhythms.

Avoiding exposure to additional toxins is also vital in supporting liver function and detox pathways. This includes minimizing the use of alcohol, tobacco, and unnecessary medications, as well as reducing exposure to environmental pollutants and chemicals found in household cleaning products, personal care items, and processed foods. Opt for natural or organic alternatives whenever possible to lessen the toxin load on your liver.

The importance of maintaining a healthy gut cannot be overstated in the context of detoxification. A well-functioning digestive system ensures that toxins are efficiently eliminated from the body, preventing their recirculation and further taxing the liver. Incorporating probiotic-rich foods such as yogurt, kefir, and fermented vegetables into your diet can help maintain a healthy gut microbiome, enhancing both digestion and detoxification processes.

Lastly, regular monitoring and testing can provide valuable insights into liver health and function. Liver function tests, available through healthcare providers, can help track the effectiveness of your detoxification efforts and identify any areas that may require additional support. These tests typically measure levels of liver enzymes, bilirubin, and proteins in the blood, offering a snapshot of liver performance and overall health.

By adopting these strategies, individuals can significantly enhance their liver's ability to detoxify from mold exposure and other toxins, leading to improved health and vitality. It's essential to approach liver support as a comprehensive lifestyle adjustment, incorporating dietary, physical, and mental health practices to fully support the body's natural detoxification processes.

7.2: Nutritional Strategies for Detoxification

To further enhance the body's resilience against the adverse effects of mold exposure, incorporating specific **nutritional strategies** is paramount. A well-structured diet plan not only supports the detoxification process but also replenishes the body with essential nutrients lost during the exposure to mold and its toxins. The following recommendations aim to provide a comprehensive approach to nutritional detoxification, emphasizing foods that are known for their potent detoxifying properties.

Antioxidant-Rich Foods: Antioxidants play a crucial role in neutralizing free radicals, thereby reducing oxidative stress and aiding in the repair of cellular damage caused by toxins. Foods high in antioxidants include berries (such as blueberries, strawberries, and raspberries), nuts (especially almonds and walnuts), dark green vegetables (like spinach, kale, and broccoli), and fruits rich in vitamin C (such as oranges, kiwis, and grapefruits). Integrating these foods into your daily diet can significantly enhance your body's natural detoxification capabilities.

Anti-Inflammatory Foods: Chronic inflammation can exacerbate the symptoms of mold toxicity, making it essential to include anti-inflammatory foods in your diet. Omega-3 fatty acids, found in fatty fish (like salmon, mackerel, and sardines), flaxseeds, chia seeds, and walnuts, are known for their anti-inflammatory properties. Additionally, turmeric and ginger are potent anti-inflammatory spices that can be easily incorporated into meals to help reduce inflammation throughout the body.

Fiber-Rich Foods: Adequate fiber intake is critical for maintaining a healthy digestive system, which is vital for the efficient elimination of toxins. Foods high in fiber, such as legumes (beans, lentils, chickpeas), whole grains (oats, quinoa, barley), fruits (apples, pears, avocados), and vegetables (carrots, beets, broccoli), help promote regular bowel movements and support the body's natural detoxification processes.

Hydration: Proper hydration is essential for detoxification, as it facilitates the elimination of toxins through urine and sweat. Drinking filtered water throughout the day is recommended to ensure the body remains adequately hydrated. Herbal teas, such as dandelion or milk thistle tea, can also be beneficial due to their diuretic and liver-supporting properties.

Probiotic and Fermented Foods: A healthy gut microbiome is crucial for detoxification and overall health. Probiotic and fermented foods, such as yogurt, kefir, sauerkraut, kimchi, and kombucha, introduce beneficial bacteria into the digestive system, aiding in digestion and the elimination of toxins.

Sulfur-Rich Foods: Sulfur plays a key role in the body's detoxification pathways, particularly in the liver. Foods high in sulfur, such as garlic, onions, leeks, and cruciferous vegetables (broccoli, Brussels sprouts, cabbage), help enhance the liver's ability to process and eliminate toxins.

Avoid Processed Foods and Sugars: Minimizing the intake of processed foods, artificial sweeteners, and refined sugars is crucial during detoxification. These foods can increase inflammation, disrupt gut health, and hinder the body's detoxification efforts. Opting for whole, unprocessed foods ensures that your body receives the highest quality nutrients without the added chemicals and preservatives.

Limit Alcohol and Caffeine: Reducing the consumption of alcohol and caffeine can significantly support the detoxification process. Both substances can place additional stress on the liver and hinder its ability to process toxins effectively.

Implementing these nutritional strategies can significantly aid in the detoxification process, helping to alleviate the symptoms of mold toxicity and restore overall health and vitality. It's important to remember that dietary changes should be introduced gradually and tailored to your individual health needs and preferences. Consulting with a healthcare professional or a registered dietitian can provide personalized guidance and ensure that your diet supports your detoxification goals.

7.3: Key Supplements and Herbs for Mold Recovery

For individuals navigating the path to recovery from mold exposure, the integration of **specific supplements and herbs** can significantly enhance the detoxification process. These compounds have been identified for their potent abilities to support the body's natural detox pathways, aid in the elimination of toxins, and bolster the immune system's response to mold-related illnesses.

Glutathione is often referred to as the body's "master antioxidant." It plays a critical role in protecting cells from oxidative stress and aiding in the detoxification of harmful substances. Supplementation with glutathione, or its precursors such as N-acetylcysteine (NAC), can help increase the body's levels of this vital antioxidant, promoting the elimination of mycotoxins and supporting overall cellular health.

Quercetin, a natural flavonoid found in many fruits and vegetables, has been shown to have powerful anti-inflammatory and antioxidant properties. It can help stabilize mast cells, reducing the release of histamine and other inflammatory substances in the body. This action can be particularly beneficial for individuals experiencing heightened sensitivity and allergic reactions due to mold exposure.

Vitamin D is crucial for immune system function, and many individuals with chronic illnesses, including those affected by mold toxicity, have been found to have low levels of this vitamin. Supplementation with vitamin D can help modulate the immune response, reducing inflammation and supporting the body's ability to fight off infections and heal from mold exposure.

Omega-3 fatty acids, found in high concentrations in fish oil, have been extensively studied for their anti-inflammatory effects. These essential fatty acids can help reduce the systemic inflammation associated with mold exposure and support cognitive function, which is often compromised in individuals suffering from mold-related health issues.

Probiotics play a vital role in maintaining gut health, which is paramount for individuals recovering from mold toxicity. The gut microbiome can be significantly impacted by mold exposure, leading to dysbiosis and a host of digestive issues. Supplementing with high-quality probiotics can help restore the balance of beneficial bacteria in the gut, enhancing digestion, nutrient absorption, and the elimination of toxins.

Milk Thistle is renowned for its liver-protective properties. The active compound in milk thistle, silymarin, has antioxidant, antiviral, and anti-inflammatory properties, making it an excellent supplement for supporting liver health and detoxification pathways.

Turmeric, containing the active compound curcumin, is another potent anti-inflammatory herb that can aid in the detoxification process. Its ability to reduce inflammation and oxidative stress can be particularly beneficial for individuals dealing with chronic illnesses and sensitivities due to mold exposure.

Activated Charcoal and **Bentonite Clay** are adsorbents that can bind to toxins in the gastrointestinal tract, preventing their absorption and facilitating their elimination from the body. These supplements can be useful in the acute phase of detoxification, helping to quickly reduce the burden of circulating mycotoxins.

Andrographis, an herb widely used in traditional Chinese and Ayurvedic medicine, has been shown to have antimicrobial, anti-inflammatory, and immune-stimulating properties. It can be particularly helpful in combating infections and supporting the immune system during the recovery from mold exposure.

Incorporating these supplements and herbs into a comprehensive detoxification protocol can offer significant benefits to individuals recovering from mold toxicity. However, it's important to consult with a healthcare professional before starting any new supplement regimen, especially for those with pre-existing health conditions or those taking other medications, to avoid potential interactions and ensure the most effective and safe approach to detoxification.

7.4: Sauna and Sweating for Detox

Infrared saunas have become a cornerstone in the detoxification process, especially for individuals recovering from mold exposure. The deep penetration of infrared heat into the body's tissues induces a more profound sweating response compared to traditional saunas. This enhanced sweating is not merely a mechanism for cooling the body but serves as a vital route for expelling a wide array of toxins, including heavy metals and, importantly, mycotoxins associated with mold illness. The effectiveness of infrared saunas lies in their ability to operate at lower, more tolerable temperatures than conventional saunas, making them accessible to a broader range of individuals, including those who may not tolerate the intense heat of standard saunas due to health issues.

The process of sweating in an infrared sauna is a gentle yet powerful method of detoxification. As the body's core temperature gradually increases, blood circulation accelerates, and the body's natural detoxification process is stimulated. This increased circulation allows the blood to carry essential nutrients to vital organs while simultaneously removing waste products. The sweat produced during a sauna session contains toxins that have been mobilized from their storage sites and are being excreted through the skin, reducing the burden on the liver and kidneys, which are the primary organs involved in detoxification.

To maximize the benefits of sauna use for detoxification, hydration is key. Drinking ample water before, during, and after sauna sessions ensures that the body can produce sufficient sweat to eliminate toxins effectively. Additionally, replenishing electrolytes lost through sweating is crucial to maintain the body's electrolyte balance and prevent dehydration. Natural sources of electrolytes, such as coconut water or electrolyte-replenishing drinks without added sugars, can be beneficial.

Another aspect to consider when incorporating sauna therapy into a detoxification protocol is the timing and frequency of sessions. Starting with shorter sessions and gradually increasing the duration allows the body to adjust to the heat stress and enhances the body's ability to detoxify over time. A general recommendation is to begin with sessions of 10 to 15 minutes, gradually increasing to 30 minutes, depending on individual tolerance and response. Consistency is crucial, with optimal results observed with regular use, typically around three to four times a week.

While infrared saunas are a valuable tool in the detoxification process, it's essential to approach their use with caution, especially for individuals with certain health conditions. Consulting with a healthcare provider before beginning sauna therapy is advisable to ensure it's appropriate based on individual health status. For those with cardiovascular issues, blood pressure concerns, or pregnant women, alternative detoxification methods may be recommended.

In addition to infrared sauna use, other methods of encouraging sweating and toxin elimination include engaging in regular, moderate-intensity exercise and utilizing steam baths. These activities also promote sweating and can complement the detoxification benefits of infrared saunas. However, the unique advantage of infrared sauna therapy lies in its ability to deeply penetrate tissues, mobilize toxins, and promote their elimination in a way that is both effective and gentle on the body.

Incorporating sauna therapy into a comprehensive detoxification strategy offers a synergistic effect when combined with nutritional support, hydration, and other detoxification methods. This holistic approach supports the body's natural detoxification pathways, aiding in the recovery from mold exposure and contributing to overall health and well-being. As with any detoxification method, individual experiences may vary, and personalization of the approach is key to achieving the best outcomes.

Chapter 8: Healing Your Systems

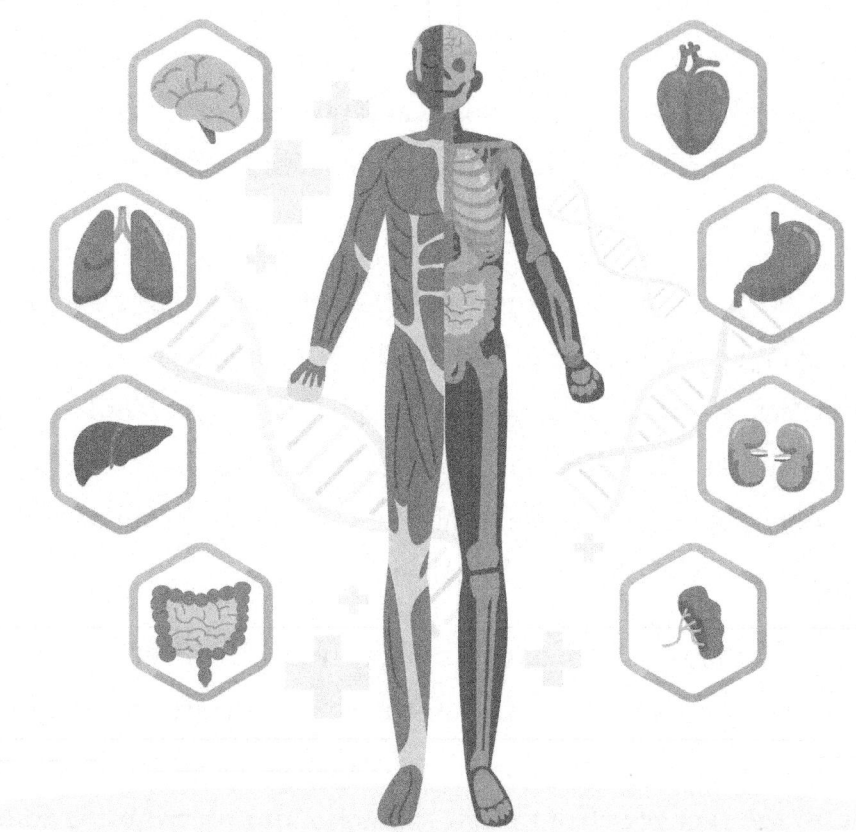

Exposure to toxic mold can wreak havoc on the body's systems, leading to a cascade of health issues that can be both perplexing and debilitating. The insidious nature of mold-related illnesses often stems from the body's multifaceted response to the invasion of mycotoxins, which can affect everything from the gut to the immune system. Understanding the breadth of damage caused by mold is the first step toward healing, and this chapter aims to shed light on the intricate ways in which mold toxicity can undermine one's health.

The gut, often referred to as the body's second brain, is particularly vulnerable to the effects of mold exposure. Mycotoxins can disrupt the delicate balance of the gut microbiome, leading to a range of gastrointestinal issues such as leaky gut syndrome, where the intestinal lining becomes more permeable than normal, allowing toxins and undigested food particles to enter the bloodstream. This condition can trigger an immune response, leading to systemic inflammation and a host of other symptoms that can confound even the most experienced healthcare practitioners. Strategies to repair gut health include adopting a diet rich in anti-inflammatory foods, taking specific supplements to restore the gut lining, and eliminating foods that feed harmful bacteria and fungi.

The immune system, our body's defense mechanism against infections and diseases, can also be severely compromised by mold exposure. Mycotoxins have the capability to suppress immune function, making the body more susceptible to infections, viruses, and a plethora of autoimmune conditions. In some cases, the immune system may become hyperactive, attacking the body's own tissues in a misguided attempt to protect the body. Rebalancing the immune system requires a multifaceted approach, including optimizing nutrient intake, managing stress, and avoiding further exposure to mold and other toxins.

Furthermore, the nervous system can suffer significantly from mold toxicity. Individuals exposed to mold may experience neurological symptoms such as headaches, memory loss, difficulty concentrating, and mood swings. These symptoms occur as a result of mycotoxins' ability to cross the blood-brain barrier, causing inflammation and oxidative stress within the brain. Approaches to support the nervous system include engaging in activities that promote neuroplasticity, such as cognitive exercises, as well as incorporating anti-inflammatory nutrients into one's diet to help mitigate the effects of oxidative stress.

As we delve deeper into the mechanisms through which mold affects these critical bodily systems, it becomes evident that the path to recovery is not linear. Each individual's

Chapter 8: Healing Your Systems

experience with mold toxicity is unique, necessitating personalized strategies for detoxification and healing. The following sections will continue to explore the specific interventions and lifestyle modifications that can support the body's journey back to health, focusing on practical steps to detoxify, heal, and restore vitality without concluding remarks or summarization.

To effectively address the hormonal and endocrine disruptions caused by mold exposure, it's crucial to understand the intricate relationship between toxins and hormonal balance. Mycotoxins can interfere with hormone production and regulation, leading to a myriad of symptoms such as fatigue, weight fluctuations, and mood disorders. Supporting the endocrine system involves a comprehensive approach that includes dietary adjustments to reduce inflammation and stabilize blood sugar levels, targeted supplementation to replenish nutrient deficiencies, and lifestyle interventions aimed at reducing stress, which can exacerbate hormonal imbalances.

Detoxification plays a pivotal role in mitigating the effects of mold exposure on the body's systems. A key strategy for detoxification involves enhancing the body's natural elimination processes through hydration, dietary fiber, and activities that promote sweating, such as exercise and sauna use. Additionally, certain supplements and herbs, specifically chosen for their ability to bind to and facilitate the removal of mycotoxins, can be invaluable. These might include activated charcoal, bentonite clay, and specific compounds known for their detoxifying properties.

Repairing the damage caused by mold exposure extends beyond physical health, encompassing emotional and mental well-being. The psychological impact of chronic illness can be profound, leading to stress, anxiety, and depression. Addressing these aspects is essential for a holistic recovery. Techniques such as mindfulness meditation, deep breathing exercises, and engaging in supportive therapy can provide significant benefits, helping individuals navigate the emotional challenges associated with healing from mold toxicity.

Preventing future exposure to mold is equally important in the healing journey. This involves identifying potential sources of mold in the environment and taking steps to mitigate these risks. Regular cleaning, using dehumidifiers in damp areas, ensuring adequate ventilation, and choosing mold-resistant materials during home repairs or renovations can all contribute to a healthier living space. Additionally, being vigilant about signs of water damage or mold growth and addressing these issues promptly can prevent the recurrence of mold-related health problems.

In summary, healing from mold toxicity requires a comprehensive and personalized approach that addresses the multifaceted nature of mold-related illnesses. By focusing on gut health, immune system support, nervous system care, hormonal balance, and detoxification, individuals can embark on a path toward restoring their health and vitality. Embracing a holistic perspective that includes both physical and emotional healing, along with preventive measures to avoid future exposure, offers the best chance for a full recovery.

8.1: Rebooting Your Nervous System

Mold exposure can lead to a variety of neurological symptoms due to the ability of mycotoxins to penetrate the blood-brain barrier, causing inflammation and oxidative stress in the brain. This can manifest as headaches, memory loss, difficulty concentrating, and mood swings. To address these challenges and support the nervous system, it's essential to adopt strategies that promote neuroplasticity and reduce inflammation.

Diet plays a crucial role in mitigating the effects of oxidative stress. Incorporating anti-inflammatory foods such as leafy greens, berries, nuts, and seeds, which are rich in antioxidants, can help protect brain cells from damage. Omega-3 fatty acids, found in fish like salmon and in flaxseeds, are particularly beneficial for brain health, supporting cognitive function and mood regulation.

Hydration is another key aspect of supporting the nervous system. Adequate water intake helps flush out toxins from the body and can improve energy levels and cognitive function. Aim for at least eight glasses of water a day, more if you are engaging in activities that cause you to sweat.

Supplementation can also play a supportive role. Certain supplements, such as magnesium, have been shown to have a calming effect on the nervous system and can aid in reducing anxiety and improving sleep quality. B vitamins, particularly B12, are crucial for maintaining healthy nerve cells and can help improve energy levels and cognitive function. Always consult with a healthcare provider before starting any new supplement regimen to ensure it's appropriate for your specific health needs.

Engaging in cognitive exercises can help improve brain function and promote neuroplasticity. Activities such as puzzles, memory games, or learning a new skill can stimulate the brain and help counteract the cognitive symptoms associated with mold exposure.

Stress management techniques such as mindfulness meditation, deep breathing exercises, and yoga can also be beneficial. Stress can exacerbate neurological symptoms, so finding effective ways to manage stress is crucial for those recovering from mold exposure. These practices not only help reduce stress but also promote overall well-being and can improve sleep quality.

Sleep quality is vital for brain health. Poor sleep can worsen neurological symptoms and impede the body's ability to detoxify. Establishing a regular sleep schedule, creating a restful environment, and avoiding stimulants before bedtime can help improve sleep quality.

Physical activity is another important component of supporting the nervous system. Regular exercise can help reduce inflammation, improve mood, and enhance cognitive function. Choose activities that you enjoy and that do not overexert the body, such as walking, swimming, or gentle yoga.

Environmental modifications may also be necessary to reduce exposure to mold and other toxins that can further stress the nervous system. This includes using air purifiers, ensuring proper ventilation, and addressing any sources of moisture or water damage in the home.

By incorporating these strategies, individuals recovering from mold exposure can support their nervous system, reduce symptoms, and promote overall healing. It's important to approach recovery with patience and to work closely with healthcare professionals to develop a personalized plan that addresses your specific needs and symptoms.

8.2: Restoring Immune Balance

To bolster the immune system following exposure to mold, it is essential to focus on **nutrient optimization**. This involves consuming a diet rich in vitamins, minerals, and antioxidants that can help combat the oxidative stress and inflammation caused by mycotoxins. Foods high in vitamin C, such as citrus fruits, berries, and leafy greens, are powerful antioxidants that support immune function. Vitamin D, obtained from sunlight exposure and fortified foods, plays a critical role in modulating the immune response and enhancing the body's defense mechanisms against pathogens.

Probiotics are another crucial component in restoring immune balance. These beneficial bacteria, found in fermented foods like yogurt, kefir, and sauerkraut, help maintain a healthy gut microbiome, which is vital for immune system health. The gut is often referred to as the body's second brain and is a significant immune organ; thus, nurturing gut health is paramount in recovering from mold toxicity.

Omega-3 fatty acids, found in fish oil, flaxseeds, and walnuts, are known for their anti-inflammatory properties. Incorporating these fats into your diet can help reduce systemic inflammation and support immune function. Similarly, foods rich in zinc, such as pumpkin seeds, beef, and spinach, can enhance immune cell activity and overall immune health.

Adequate hydration is essential for lymphatic drainage and the elimination of toxins from the body. Drinking sufficient amounts of water daily helps keep the immune system functioning optimally by assisting in the production of lymph, which carries white blood cells and other immune system cells.

Regular, moderate exercise can boost the immune system by promoting good circulation, which allows the cells and substances of the immune system to move through the body freely and do their job efficiently. However, it's crucial to balance activity levels, as excessive exercise can lead to immune suppression, especially in those recovering from mold exposure.

Stress reduction techniques, such as meditation, yoga, and deep breathing exercises, can significantly impact immune health. Chronic stress can suppress immune function, so finding effective ways to manage stress is essential in restoring immune balance. These practices not only help reduce stress but also improve sleep quality, another critical factor in immune system health.

Sleep hygiene practices can enhance immune function. Ensuring seven to nine hours of quality sleep per night allows the body to repair and regenerate immune cells. Creating a restful environment, free from electronic devices and disturbances, can improve sleep quality.

Avoiding further exposure to mold and other toxins is crucial in preventing additional immune system stress. This may involve making changes to your living or working environment to reduce mold growth and exposure to other environmental toxins.

By implementing these strategies, individuals recovering from mold exposure can support and strengthen their immune system, aiding in the detoxification process and promoting overall health and well-being.

8.3: Repairing Gut Health After Mold Exposure

Repairing gut health after exposure to mold and its byproducts requires a targeted approach to restore the integrity of the gastrointestinal tract and rebalance the gut microbiome. Mycotoxins can severely disrupt the delicate ecosystem within the gut, leading to a cascade of health issues that extend beyond digestive discomfort. Implementing a gut-healing protocol involves several key strategies aimed at reducing inflammation, eliminating harmful pathogens, and replenishing beneficial gut flora.

Elimination of Inflammatory Foods: Begin by removing foods that contribute to inflammation and gut permeability. Common culprits include processed foods, sugars, gluten, dairy, and certain vegetable oils. These foods can exacerbate the damage caused by mycotoxins and hinder the healing process.

Incorporate Gut-Healing Foods: Focus on including foods known for their gut-healing properties. Bone broth, rich in collagen, helps repair the gut lining. Fermented foods like sauerkraut, kimchi, and kefir introduce beneficial probiotics that support a healthy microbiome. High-fiber foods, such as vegetables and legumes, promote the growth of good bacteria and aid in toxin elimination.

Supplementation for Repair and Rebalance: Certain supplements can be particularly beneficial in repairing gut health. L-glutamine, an amino acid, is essential for repairing the intestinal lining. Probiotics help replenish beneficial bacteria, while prebiotics feed those good bacteria. Omega-3 supplements can reduce inflammation throughout the body, including the gut.

Detoxification Support: Enhancing the body's natural detoxification processes is crucial in eliminating mycotoxins from the body. This can be supported through increased hydration, encouraging regular bowel movements, and incorporating detoxifying foods such as garlic, cilantro, and cruciferous vegetables.

Stress Management: Chronic stress can exacerbate gut health issues by impairing the gut barrier and altering gut bacteria. Implementing stress-reduction techniques such as yoga, meditation, and deep breathing exercises can have a positive impact on gut health.

Sleep Optimization: Quality sleep is vital for gut health. The body's repair processes are most active during sleep, including those in the gut. Establishing a regular sleep schedule and creating a restful sleeping environment can support the healing process.

Exercise: Regular, moderate exercise can improve gut health by reducing inflammation and stress. However, it's important to balance exercise intensity to avoid exacerbating any existing health issues.

Avoiding Antibiotics When Possible: Antibiotics can disrupt the gut microbiome by killing off beneficial bacteria along with harmful bacteria. If antibiotics are necessary, ensure to follow up with a course of probiotics to restore the gut flora.

Mindful Eating: Paying attention to how your body responds to different foods and adjusting your diet accordingly can help identify foods that support your gut health and those that may be detrimental.

Implementing these strategies requires patience and consistency. The damage caused by mold exposure and mycotoxins didn't occur overnight, and neither will the healing process. It's also important to work closely with healthcare professionals who can provide guidance tailored to your specific health situation. They can offer additional insights into dietary adjustments, supplement regimens, and other therapeutic interventions to support gut health and overall well-being.

8.4: Managing Hormonal and Endocrine Disruptions

Mold exposure can lead to significant disruptions in the endocrine system, which regulates hormones critical for maintaining balance in nearly every physiological process in the body. When mycotoxins from mold enter the body, they can mimic, block, or disrupt the normal function of hormones, leading to a wide range of health issues, from thyroid dysfunction to adrenal fatigue. To address these disruptions and restore hormonal balance, a multifaceted approach is necessary, focusing on diet, supplementation, stress management, and lifestyle adjustments.

Dietary Adjustments for Hormonal Balance: Incorporating foods that support hormonal health is crucial. Foods rich in omega-3 fatty acids, such as wild-caught fish and flaxseeds, can help reduce inflammation, which is often a precursor to hormonal imbalances. Cruciferous vegetables like broccoli and Brussels sprouts contain indole-3-carbinol, which helps in the detoxification of estrogen and can be beneficial for maintaining estrogen balance. Additionally, foods high in fiber support the elimination of excess hormones through the digestive tract, aiding in overall hormonal balance.

Supplementation to Support the Endocrine System: Certain supplements can be particularly beneficial in addressing hormonal disruptions caused by mold exposure. Adaptogenic herbs such as ashwagandha, rhodiola, and holy basil can help modulate the body's stress response, supporting adrenal health and cortisol balance. Magnesium, often depleted during times of stress, is vital for hundreds of biochemical reactions in the body, including those that regulate hormonal activity. Vitamin D and selenium are also critical for thyroid function and can help support the body's natural hormone production.

Stress Management Techniques: Chronic stress can exacerbate hormonal imbalances by taxing the adrenal glands and disrupting cortisol levels, which in turn affects other hormones such as insulin, estrogen, and progesterone. Implementing stress management techniques such as mindfulness meditation, deep breathing exercises, and gentle yoga can help reduce the body's stress response and support hormonal balance.

Lifestyle Adjustments for Detoxification and Healing: Reducing exposure to environmental toxins, including mold, is essential for allowing the endocrine system to recover. Using air purifiers, ensuring proper ventilation, and addressing any water damage or mold growth in living spaces can help minimize further exposure. Regular exercise helps to boost detoxification through sweat and supports overall metabolic health, which is closely linked to hormonal balance. Ensuring adequate sleep is also crucial, as sleep deprivation can severely impact hormonal health, particularly the regulation of cortisol, growth hormone, and insulin.

Monitoring and Adjusting: Healing from mold-induced hormonal disruptions is an ongoing process that requires monitoring and adjustments. Working with healthcare professionals who can provide personalized advice and adjustments based on lab tests and symptom tracking is essential. Regular testing can help track the progress of hormonal rebalancing efforts and guide the adjustment of dietary, supplement, and lifestyle strategies to ensure optimal results.

By addressing hormonal and endocrine disruptions with targeted dietary, supplemental, stress management, and lifestyle interventions, individuals recovering from mold exposure can take significant steps toward restoring their health and vitality. This comprehensive approach supports the body's natural healing processes, helping to rebalance the endocrine system and alleviate the wide range of symptoms associated with mold-induced hormonal imbalances.

Part 4:
Co-Infections and Chronic Illness

Chapter 9: Lyme Disease and Mold Toxicity

9.1: Mold and Lyme Symptom Overlap

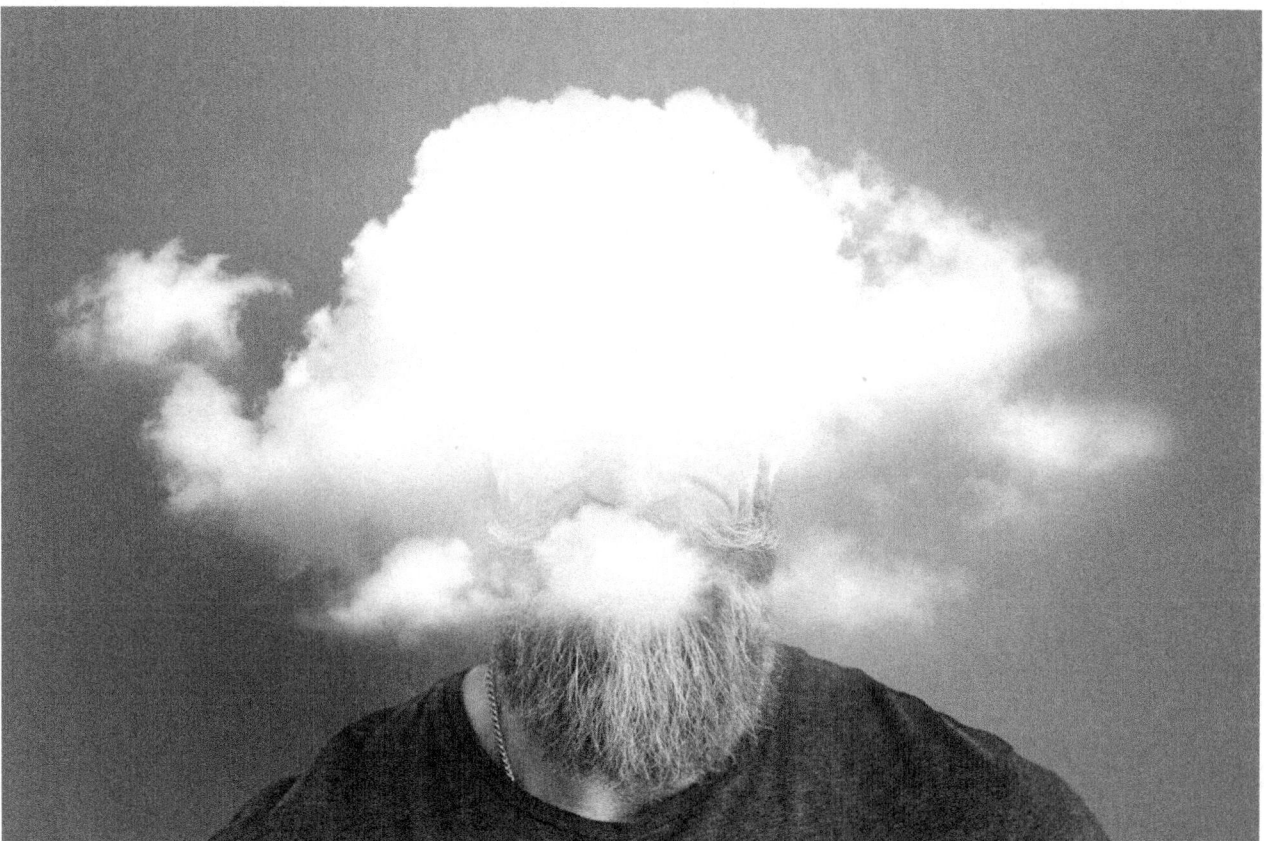

Fatigue, brain fog, and joint pain are hallmark symptoms that both mold toxicity and Lyme disease share, creating a complex web of overlapping signs that can confound even the most astute healthcare practitioners. The intricacies of these conditions mean that individuals may suffer from a wide array of symptoms that are not only debilitating but also remarkably similar, making the differentiation between mold exposure and Lyme disease a challenging endeavor.

Fatigue in the context of mold toxicity and Lyme disease is not just a mere feeling of tiredness; it is a profound exhaustion that does not improve with rest. This type of fatigue can severely impact an individual's daily functioning, making even simple tasks seem insurmountable. The underlying cause is multifaceted, involving the body's attempt to fight off toxins or infections, leading to an overtaxed immune system that can no longer sustain normal energy levels.

Brain fog, another shared symptom, manifests as cognitive impairments that can range from mild forgetfulness to severe difficulties in concentration and decision-making. Individuals may experience a sense of disorientation, struggling to process information or recall basic facts. This cognitive decline is linked to the inflammatory responses triggered by both mold mycotoxins and the bacteria responsible for Lyme disease, which can disrupt normal brain function and neurotransmitter activity.

Joint pain, often fluctuating and migrating from one joint to another, is a common complaint among those affected by either condition. The pain can be sharp and debilitating or present as a dull, persistent ache. In mold toxicity, the pain is primarily due to the inflammatory response elicited by mycotoxins, while in Lyme disease, it is caused by the body's reaction to the Borrelia burgdorferi bacteria. Both pathogens can lead to an immune system overreaction, resulting in joint inflammation and discomfort.

Understanding the overlap in symptoms between mold toxicity and Lyme disease is crucial for developing effective treatment strategies. It necessitates a comprehensive approach that addresses not only the eradication of mold and the treatment of Lyme disease but also the management of the body's inflammatory response and support for the immune system. Strategies may include dietary modifications to reduce inflammation, supplements to support detoxification and immune function, and medications or herbal remedies specifically targeted at treating Lyme disease or mold toxicity.

In conclusion, the shared symptoms of fatigue, brain fog, and joint pain highlight the complex relationship between mold toxicity and Lyme disease. Recognizing these overlaps is the first step in unraveling the complexities of these conditions, paving the way for targeted interventions that can alleviate symptoms and restore health. As we continue to explore the connections between environmental toxins and chronic illnesses, it becomes increasingly clear that a holistic and integrative approach to health is essential for those seeking to overcome the challenges posed by mold toxicity and Lyme disease.

9.2: Treating Lyme and Mold Toxicity Together

When tackling the dual challenge of Lyme disease and mold toxicity, a multifaceted approach is essential to address both conditions effectively and maximize recovery. The complexity of these illnesses requires a strategy that not only focuses on eradicating the underlying infections and exposures but also supports the body's healing and detoxification processes.

Firstly, it is critical to establish a clear diagnosis for both Lyme disease and mold toxicity. This involves comprehensive testing that can identify the presence of Lyme bacteria, co-infections, and mycotoxins in the body. Once a diagnosis is confirmed, a personalized treatment plan can be developed, taking into consideration the unique aspects of each individual's condition.

Secondly, antibiotic therapy is often a cornerstone of Lyme disease treatment, aimed at eliminating the Borrelia burgdorferi bacteria. However, when mold toxicity is also a factor, care must be taken to support the body's detoxification pathways to handle the additional burden of mycotoxins. This may involve the use of binders that can absorb and facilitate the removal of toxins from the body, alongside antibiotics.

Thirdly, addressing the inflammatory response is crucial in both conditions. Anti-inflammatory diets, rich in fruits, vegetables, healthy fats, and lean proteins, can help reduce systemic inflammation. Supplements such as omega-3 fatty acids, turmeric, and ginger may also be beneficial in managing inflammation. Reducing inflammation not only alleviates symptoms but also supports overall immune function.

Fourthly, supporting the immune system is paramount. Both Lyme disease and mold exposure can significantly weaken the immune response, making it harder for the body to fight infections and toxins. Nutritional supplements, including vitamin C, vitamin D, zinc, and selenium, can bolster the immune system. Probiotics and prebiotics are also essential in maintaining a healthy gut microbiome, which plays a critical role in immune health.

Fifthly, detoxification strategies extend beyond dietary changes and supplements. Practices such as infrared sauna sessions, dry brushing, and Epsom salt baths can support the body's natural detoxification processes through the skin. Adequate hydration is also vital to help flush toxins from the body.

Sixthly, addressing environmental factors is essential for long-term recovery. This means ensuring that the living and working environments are free from mold and other potential triggers. Regular inspections, moisture control, and air purification can help maintain a healthy indoor environment.

Seventhly, managing stress and supporting mental health are important aspects of recovery. Chronic illness can take a significant toll on emotional well-being. Techniques such as mindfulness meditation, yoga, and counseling can provide valuable support, reducing stress and improving quality of life.

Eighthly, sleep optimization plays a critical role in healing. Both Lyme disease and mold toxicity can disrupt sleep patterns, compromising the body's ability to recover. Establishing a regular sleep schedule, creating a restful sleep environment, and possibly using natural sleep aids can help improve sleep quality.

Lastly, regular follow-up with healthcare providers is necessary to monitor progress, adjust treatment plans as needed, and address any emerging issues. Recovery from Lyme disease and mold toxicity can be a long and challenging process, requiring ongoing support and adjustments to treatment strategies.

By adopting a comprehensive and personalized approach that addresses the complexities of Lyme disease and mold toxicity, individuals can work towards recovery and the restoration of their health. It is important to work closely with healthcare professionals who understand the intricacies of these conditions and can provide guidance tailored to each person's unique needs.

9.3 Managing Co-Infections: Bartonella, Babesia

Bartonella and Babesia are two of the most common co-infections in individuals suffering from Lyme disease, each bringing its unique set of challenges to the already complex symptomatology associated with mold toxicity. Bartonella, often referred to as "cat scratch fever," can cause a wide range of symptoms, including fever, fatigue, headache, poor appetite, and an unusual streaked rash that resembles stretch marks. Babesia, on the other hand, is a malaria-like parasite that infects red blood cells, leading to symptoms such as high fever, chills, sweats, fatigue, and jaundice. The interaction between these co-infections and mold toxicity can exacerbate the body's inflammatory response, complicate the clinical picture, and hinder the recovery process.

Managing these co-infections requires a nuanced understanding of their lifecycle and their ability to evade the immune system. For Bartonella, antibiotics such as doxycycline or rifampin are often used, but their effectiveness can be limited by the pathogen's intracellular location. Enhancing the body's immune response through nutritional support and supplements like omega-3 fatty acids, probiotics, and antioxidants can be beneficial. Babesia treatment typically involves a combination of antimicrobial agents like atovaquone plus azithromycin, aiming to eradicate the parasite from the bloodstream. However, due to the complexity of Babesia and its resistance to treatment, a longer course of therapy may be necessary, along with supportive treatments to manage symptoms and improve immune function.

The role of detoxification in managing these co-infections cannot be overstated. Toxins produced by mold and the pathogens themselves can overwhelm the body's detox pathways, leading to an accumulation of harmful substances that exacerbate symptoms. Supporting liver function with milk thistle, N-acetylcysteine (NAC), and glutathione, alongside regular use of detoxification practices like infrared sauna and dry brushing, can help in reducing the toxic burden. Additionally, ensuring adequate hydration and fiber intake will facilitate the elimination of toxins through urine and feces.

Dietary modifications play a crucial role in managing the inflammatory response associated with both Lyme co-infections and mold toxicity. A diet rich in anti-inflammatory foods such as leafy green vegetables, berries, omega-3-rich fish, and turmeric can help reduce systemic inflammation. Simultaneously, reducing sugar and processed foods minimizes the food source for harmful bacteria and fungi, potentially lowering the pathogenic load.

Immune system support is paramount, as both Bartonella and Babesia can suppress the immune response, making it difficult for the body to fight off these infections and mold toxicity. Vitamin D, zinc, selenium, and vitamin C are critical for immune function and can help bolster the body's defenses. Herbal remedies like astragalus, echinacea, and cat's claw may also support immune health, though it's important to consult with a healthcare provider to ensure they're appropriate for your situation.

Addressing environmental factors is essential for long-term management. Reducing exposure to mold by ensuring clean, dry, and well-ventilated living conditions can help decrease the body's toxic load. Regularly inspecting the home for signs of mold and addressing any issues promptly can prevent further exposure and support recovery from both Lyme disease and its co-infections.

In managing Bartonella, Babesia, and other Lyme co-infections alongside mold toxicity, a comprehensive approach that includes medical treatment, nutritional support, detoxification, and environmental modifications is crucial. Collaboration with a knowledgeable healthcare provider who understands the complexities of these conditions can guide the development of an effective treatment plan tailored to the individual's needs. Through diligent management and support, it is possible to mitigate the effects of these co-infections, reduce symptoms, and move towards recovery.

Chapter 10: Chronic Illness and Mold

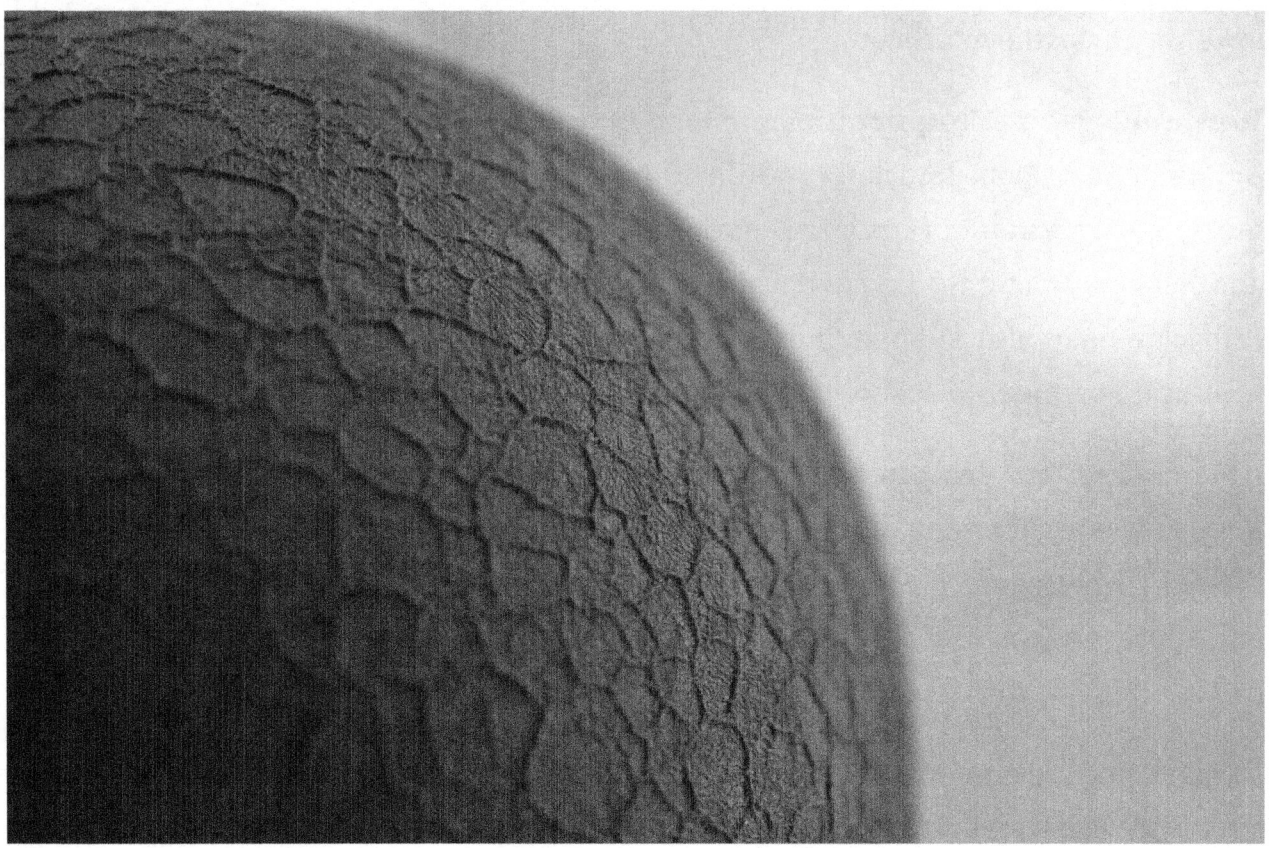

10.1: Mold and Autoimmune Disorders

Mold exposure can lead to autoimmune disorders through several mechanisms, fundamentally altering the body's immune response. When mold spores are inhaled or come into contact with the skin, they can introduce mycotoxins and other antigens into the body. These foreign substances can trigger an immune response, which, in a healthy system, helps to eliminate the invaders. However, in some individuals, this response can become dysregulated, leading to an autoimmune process where the body mistakenly attacks its own tissues.

Mycotoxins, the toxic compounds produced by certain molds, are particularly adept at disrupting normal immune function. They can bind to DNA, RNA, and proteins within human cells, causing direct damage and leading to the production of autoantibodies. These autoantibodies target the body's own cells, mistaking them for foreign invaders. This process can initiate and exacerbate autoimmune diseases such as Hashimoto's thyroiditis, where the immune system attacks the thyroid gland, or lupus, which can affect the skin, joints, and organs.

Chronic inflammation is another pathway through which mold exposure contributes to autoimmune disorders. Mycotoxins can induce a persistent inflammatory response, where the body is in a constant state of fighting against perceived threats. This state of chronic inflammation can lower the threshold for the development of autoimmune diseases, as the immune system becomes hyperactive and more likely to attack healthy tissues.

Genetic predisposition plays a crucial role in determining who will develop an autoimmune disorder following mold exposure. Individuals with certain genetic markers are more susceptible to the harmful effects of mycotoxins and more likely to experience an autoimmune response. This genetic variability explains why some people can live in moldy environments without apparent ill effects, while others may develop serious health issues.

Gut health is significantly impacted by mold exposure, which in turn affects immune regulation. The gut microbiome, a complex community of microorganisms living in the digestive tract, plays a critical role in educating and regulating the immune system. Mycotoxins can alter the composition of the gut microbiome, leading to increased intestinal permeability, also known as leaky gut syndrome. This condition allows toxins, undigested food particles, and other antigens to pass through the gut lining into the bloodstream, where they can trigger an autoimmune response.

To address the risk of autoimmune disorders following mold exposure, it is essential to:

- **Reduce exposure to mold** by identifying and eliminating mold sources in the environment. This may involve professional mold remediation and regular monitoring of indoor air quality.

- **Support detoxification pathways** to help the body eliminate mycotoxins. This can include dietary changes, supplements that enhance liver function, and practices such as sauna therapy to promote sweating.

- **Manage inflammation** through a diet rich in anti-inflammatory foods, regular physical activity, and stress reduction techniques. Anti-inflammatory supplements, such as omega-3 fatty acids and turmeric, may also be beneficial.

- **Support gut health** with a diet high in fiber, fermented foods, and probiotics to help restore a healthy gut microbiome. Supplements like L-glutamine may also help repair the gut lining.

- **Consult with healthcare professionals** who are knowledgeable about mold exposure and autoimmune diseases to develop a personalized treatment plan. This may include testing for mycotoxins, autoimmune markers, and gut health assessments to guide interventions.

By understanding the mechanisms through which mold exposure can trigger autoimmune disorders, individuals can take proactive steps to protect their health and mitigate the risk of developing conditions like Hashimoto's or lupus.

10.2: Mold's Role in Chronic Fatigue and Fibromyalgia

Chronic Fatigue Syndrome (CFS) and Fibromyalgia (FM) are conditions characterized by widespread pain, fatigue, and a host of other symptoms that significantly impact the quality of life. The connection between these conditions and mold exposure is increasingly recognized, shedding light on the importance of environmental factors in the management and treatment of CFS and FM. Mold exposure can trigger an array of biochemical disruptions in the body, leading to symptoms that overlap significantly with those of CFS and FM. This includes immune dysregulation, chronic inflammation, and neuroendocrine abnormalities, which are central to the symptomatology of both conditions.

Immune Dysregulation: Mold spores and mycotoxins can compromise the immune system, leading to an imbalanced immune response. In individuals with CFS and FM, this can exacerbate symptoms such as fatigue, malaise, and susceptibility to infections. Supporting the immune system through targeted nutritional supplements, such as Vitamin D, Vitamin C, and zinc, alongside a diet rich in antioxidants and phytonutrients, can help mitigate this dysregulation.

Chronic Inflammation: Mycotoxins are potent triggers of inflammatory pathways in the body. This inflammation can manifest as joint pain, muscle aches, and widespread discomfort, closely mirroring the pain experienced by individuals with FM. Anti-inflammatory strategies, including omega-3 fatty acids, turmeric, and a diet low in processed foods and high in fruits and vegetables, are crucial in managing this aspect.

Neuroendocrine Abnormalities: Exposure to mold can also affect the hypothalamic-pituitary-adrenal (HPA) axis, leading to alterations in cortisol levels and circadian rhythm. These changes can contribute to the profound fatigue and sleep disturbances common in CFS and FM. Approaches to support the HPA axis include adaptogenic herbs like ashwagandha and rhodiola, stress management techniques, and ensuring adequate sleep hygiene.

Detoxification Support: Given the role of mycotoxins in perpetuating symptoms of CFS and FM, enhancing the body's detoxification pathways is a pivotal aspect of treatment. This can be achieved through increased hydration, dietary fiber, and supplements such as milk thistle and N-acetylcysteine (NAC) to support liver function. Practices like infrared sauna use and dry brushing can further aid in the elimination of toxins through the skin.

Environmental Modifications: Minimizing mold exposure is fundamental to the recovery process. This involves identifying and addressing sources of mold in the living and working environment, using dehumidifiers to reduce indoor humidity levels, and ensuring adequate ventilation to prevent mold growth. Professional mold remediation may be necessary in cases of significant infestation.

Gut Health: The gut microbiome plays a critical role in overall health and is particularly relevant in the context of CFS and FM. Mold exposure can disrupt gut flora, leading to increased intestinal permeability and exacerbating symptoms. A diet rich in fermented foods, fiber, and the judicious use of probiotics can support gut healing and reduce systemic inflammation.

Pain Management: For individuals with FM, managing pain is a top priority. In addition to pharmaceutical options, complementary therapies such as acupuncture, massage, and gentle exercise like yoga and tai chi can be beneficial. These practices not only address pain but also contribute to stress reduction and improved sleep.

Cognitive Function: Brain fog is a common complaint among those with CFS and FM. Strategies to enhance cognitive function include ensuring adequate omega-3 intake, engaging in regular physical and mental exercise, and utilizing cognitive behavioral therapy (CBT) to develop coping strategies.

In addressing CFS and FM in the context of mold exposure, a multifaceted approach that includes medical intervention, dietary modifications, lifestyle changes, and environmental controls is essential. Collaboration with healthcare providers experienced in environmental medicine and integrative health approaches can provide individuals with a comprehensive plan tailored to their specific needs, facilitating a path toward recovery and improved quality of life.

10.3: Supporting Long-Term Recovery

Building a **support network** is pivotal in navigating the complexities of long-term recovery from chronic illness and mold exposure. This network can include healthcare providers, family, friends, and support groups that understand the intricacies of your condition. A strong support system can offer emotional encouragement, share resources, and provide practical assistance on difficult days. Additionally, engaging with online forums and local community groups can offer insights and camaraderie from those on similar paths, fostering a sense of belonging and mutual understanding.

Personalized healthcare is another cornerstone of sustained recovery. Working closely with practitioners who specialize in mold toxicity and chronic illnesses ensures that your treatment plan is tailored to your unique needs. This approach may include regular health check-ups, adjustments in medication or supplements, and ongoing assessments to monitor progress. Emphasize the importance of open communication with your healthcare team, sharing any changes in symptoms or concerns you have, to facilitate adjustments in your treatment protocol as needed.

Educational empowerment plays a crucial role in managing chronic illness. Equip yourself with knowledge about your condition, treatment options, and lifestyle adjustments that can mitigate symptoms. Reliable sources include peer-reviewed journals, reputable health websites, and books dedicated to mold toxicity and chronic illness. Understanding the science behind your condition not only helps in making informed decisions about your health but also empowers you to advocate for yourself in medical settings.

Lifestyle modifications are essential for reducing exposure to mold and supporting your body's healing process. This includes maintaining a clean, dry, and well-ventilated living environment to prevent mold growth. Use dehumidifiers, fix leaks promptly, and avoid storing items in damp areas to reduce moisture. Additionally, adopting a diet low in sugar and processed foods while rich in nutrients can support detoxification and reduce inflammation. Regular, gentle exercise tailored to your energy levels can improve physical strength and enhance mental well-being.

Stress management techniques such as mindfulness meditation, deep breathing exercises, and yoga can significantly impact your recovery by reducing stress and anxiety, which are known to exacerbate symptoms of chronic illness. Incorporating these practices into your daily routine can help in managing the psychological aspects of living with a chronic condition, promoting a more balanced and peaceful state of mind.

Quality sleep is fundamental to healing. Ensure your sleeping environment supports restorative sleep by keeping it dark, quiet, and cool. Establish a regular sleep schedule, limit exposure to screens before bedtime, and consider natural sleep aids if necessary,

Chapter 10: Chronic Illness and Mold

under the guidance of your healthcare provider. Adequate rest is crucial for the body's repair processes and can improve overall energy levels and cognitive function.

Detoxification practices remain a key component of long-term management. This can include sauna therapy, dry brushing, and lymphatic massage to support the body's natural detox pathways. Consult with a healthcare professional to determine the most appropriate detoxification strategies for your situation, and remember to stay hydrated to facilitate toxin elimination.

Ongoing education and adaptation are necessary as new research emerges and your health evolves. Stay informed about the latest developments in mold toxicity and chronic illness treatment, and be willing to adjust your approach as you learn more about what works best for your body. This proactive stance not only keeps you at the forefront of potential therapeutic options but also fosters a sense of control over your health journey.

Celebrating small victories and acknowledging progress, no matter how incremental, can boost morale and motivation. Recovery is often nonlinear, with ups and downs, but recognizing improvements in your well-being can encourage persistence and resilience. Keep a journal to document your journey, noting positive changes and reflecting on challenges overcome. This can serve as a powerful reminder of your strength and progress over time.

Incorporating these strategies into your approach to managing chronic illness and mold exposure can support a holistic and dynamic path to recovery. It's about creating a personalized framework that addresses not only the physical but also the emotional and environmental aspects of healing. By actively engaging in your recovery process, adapting strategies as needed, and leaning on your support network, you can navigate the complexities of chronic illness with confidence and hope.

Part 5:
Restoring Vitality and Preventing Relapse

Chapter 11: Emotional and Mental Healing

11.1: Coping with Stress and Anxiety

In the throes of recovery from mold toxicity and chronic illness, stress and anxiety can often serve as formidable barriers to healing. The uncertainty of the journey, coupled with the physical toll of detoxification, can exacerbate feelings of unease and worry. However, adopting effective stress management techniques can significantly alleviate these emotional burdens and foster a more conducive environment for physical and mental recovery. Here are several strategies to manage stress and anxiety during this challenging period:

1. **Practice Mindfulness and Meditation**: Engaging in mindfulness practices can help anchor you in the present moment, reducing the tendency to ruminate on past struggles or future concerns. Meditation, even for short periods daily, can lower stress levels and enhance overall well-being.

2. **Deep Breathing Exercises**: Simple yet profoundly effective, deep breathing techniques can activate the body's relaxation response, counteracting the stress response. Techniques such as the 4-7-8 method or diaphragmatic breathing can be particularly beneficial.

3. **Establish a Routine**: A structured daily routine can provide a sense of normalcy and control amidst the chaos of recovery. Incorporating regular meals, sleep schedules, and time for relaxation can stabilize your mood and reduce anxiety.

4. **Connect with Supportive Communities**: Finding a community or support group of individuals who understand what you're going through can be incredibly validating and comforting. Sharing experiences and coping strategies can lessen the feeling of isolation that often accompanies chronic illness.

5. **Engage in Gentle Physical Activity**: Exercise, tailored to your current ability and energy levels, can significantly impact stress and anxiety. Activities like walking, yoga, or tai chi can boost mood, improve sleep, and enhance your sense of well-being.

6. **Limit Stimulant Intake**: Caffeine and sugar can exacerbate anxiety and disrupt sleep patterns. Reducing or eliminating these stimulants from your diet can help stabilize your mood and improve sleep quality.

7. **Prioritize Sleep**: Quality sleep is crucial for mental health and stress management. Establishing a calming bedtime routine and creating a comfortable, dark, and cool sleep environment can improve sleep quality.

8. **Seek Professional Help**: Sometimes, the support of a therapist or counselor skilled in dealing with chronic illness and stress management can be invaluable. They can provide personalized strategies and coping mechanisms to navigate this challenging time.

9. **Journaling**: Writing down your thoughts and feelings can serve as a therapeutic outlet for your anxieties and fears. Reflecting on your writing can also help you identify patterns in your stressors and develop strategies to address them.

10. **Limit Exposure to Stressful Media**: Constant exposure to news and social media can heighten anxiety. Setting boundaries around media consumption can help maintain a more peaceful state of mind.

11. **Practice Gratitude**: Focusing on gratitude can shift your perspective from one of scarcity or loss to one of appreciation and abundance. Keeping a gratitude journal or simply reflecting on things you're thankful for each day can enhance emotional resilience.

12. **Engage in Creative Activities**: Creative expression, whether through art, music, writing, or another medium, can provide a therapeutic outlet for emotions and reduce stress.

By incorporating these strategies into your recovery process, you can create a more balanced and serene mental landscape, paving the way for more effective healing and restoration of vitality.

11.2: Reclaiming Emotional Balance

Incorporating mindfulness and relaxation techniques into your daily routine can be a transformative practice for those healing from mold toxicity and chronic illness. These methods not only aid in reducing stress and anxiety but also play a crucial role in fostering emotional balance. Here, we delve into additional practices that complement meditation and deep breathing exercises, further supporting your journey towards emotional healing.

Visualization and Guided Imagery: This technique involves focusing your mind on positive, peaceful images or scenarios to evoke feelings of relaxation. By visualizing a serene environment or a happy memory, you can shift your body's response away from stress. Engaging in guided imagery can be particularly effective before bedtime to promote restful sleep.

Progressive Muscle Relaxation (PMR): PMR is a method where you tense each muscle group in the body tightly, but not to the point of strain, and then slowly relax them. Starting from the toes and moving upwards through the body can systematically reduce physical tension and associated mental stress.

Mindful Eating: Transforming meals into mindful experiences can help reduce stress and improve your relationship with food. This involves eating slowly, savoring each bite, and paying attention to the flavors, textures, and sensations of your food. Mindful eating can enhance digestion and satisfaction with meals.

Nature Therapy: Spending time in nature, whether it's a walk in the park, gardening, or simply sitting under a tree, can have a profound calming effect. Natural settings have been shown to lower stress hormone levels, improve mood, and enhance cognitive function.

Aromatherapy: The use of essential oils, whether diffused into the air, added to bathwater, or applied topically, can provide stress relief and relaxation. Lavender, chamomile, and sandalwood are among the scents known for their calming properties.

Yoga Nidra: Also known as yogic sleep, Yoga Nidra is a state of consciousness between waking and sleeping, induced by a guided meditation. This practice is incredibly restorative, offering deep relaxation and an opportunity to release long-held tensions in the body and mind.

Digital Detox: Reducing screen time, especially before bed, can significantly improve mental health and sleep quality. Setting aside specific times to disconnect from digital devices allows your mind to unwind and can reduce the stress associated with constant connectivity.

Art Therapy: Engaging in artistic activities such as painting, drawing, or sculpting can be a powerful outlet for expressing emotions and reducing stress. Art therapy provides a distraction, allowing you to take a break from habitual thought patterns and engage in a mindful activity.

Music Therapy: Listening to music or playing an instrument can be therapeutic and calming. Music has the ability to lower blood pressure, reduce heart rate, and decrease anxiety levels. Creating a playlist of songs that bring you joy or relaxation can be a helpful tool in managing stress.

Acupressure: This technique involves applying pressure to specific points on the body to release muscle tension and promote relaxation. Acupressure can be learned and practiced at home as a method to alleviate stress and improve emotional balance.

By integrating these practices into your life, you can enhance your ability to manage stress, reduce anxiety, and support your emotional well-being. Each technique offers a unique pathway to relaxation and peace, contributing to a holistic approach to healing from mold toxicity and chronic illness.

11.3: Overcoming Chronic Illness Isolation

Building a robust support system is a cornerstone in overcoming the psychological toll of chronic illness, including the challenges posed by mold toxicity. The feeling of isolation can be profound, as friends, family, and even medical professionals may not fully understand the depth of your experience. However, fostering connections and seeking out those who can offer understanding, empathy, and practical support can significantly mitigate feelings of loneliness and misunderstanding.

Identify Allies in Your Personal Network: Start by identifying friends or family members who show an inclination to understand and support you. Educating them about your condition can turn them into allies who provide emotional support and practical help when needed. It's important to communicate openly about what you're going through and how they can assist you.

Seek Out Support Groups: Many find solace and understanding in support groups composed of individuals facing similar health challenges. These groups offer a platform to share experiences, strategies for coping, and emotional support. Online forums and social media groups can also serve as valuable resources for connecting with others who truly understand what it means to live with mold toxicity and chronic illness.

Professional Support: Consider seeking the help of a mental health professional who can guide you through the emotional challenges associated with chronic illness. Therapists or counselors experienced in chronic health conditions can offer coping strategies, therapeutic interventions, and a non-judgmental space to process your feelings.

Leverage Online Resources: The internet is a vast repository of information and support. Websites, blogs, and online communities dedicated to mold toxicity recovery can offer advice, encouragement, and a sense of belonging. Engaging with these resources can help reduce feelings of isolation and provide practical tips for managing your condition.

Volunteer or Advocate: Engaging in advocacy or volunteer work related to mold toxicity and chronic illness can provide a sense of purpose and community. Sharing your story, raising awareness, or supporting others in similar situations can be empowering and help build connections with individuals who share your concerns and goals.

Develop a Wellness Team: Building a team of healthcare providers who are knowledgeable about mold toxicity and sympathetic to your journey is crucial. This team may include medical doctors, naturopaths, nutritionists, and other specialists who understand the complexities of mold-related illnesses and can offer comprehensive care.

Cultivate Self-Compassion: It's essential to practice self-compassion and kindness towards yourself during this challenging time. Recognize that feeling isolated or misunderstood is a common experience among those with chronic illnesses, and it's okay to seek help and support.

Maintain Hobbies and Interests: Engaging in hobbies and activities that bring you joy can provide a distraction from illness and foster connections with others who share your interests. Whether it's art, music, gardening, or another pastime, maintaining these interests can offer a sense of normalcy and fulfillment.

Set Boundaries: Learning to set healthy boundaries with people who may not understand or respect your experience is important. It's okay to limit your time with individuals who drain your energy or dismiss your feelings. Prioritizing relationships that uplift and support you is crucial for your emotional well-being.

Practice Effective Communication: Developing the skills to effectively communicate your needs and experiences can enhance your relationships and support system. Be clear about what you're going through and how others can help, but also be open to listening and appreciating the support offered.

By actively building and nurturing a support system, you can alleviate the emotional burden of feeling isolated or misunderstood. Remember, reaching out for help is a sign of strength, and connecting with others who understand your journey can provide immense comfort and encouragement as you navigate the path to recovery.

Chapter 12: Rebuilding Energy and Vitality

12.1: Nutritional Strategies to Regain Energy

Incorporating specific **nutrients** into your diet can play a pivotal role in regaining energy and repairing cellular damage caused by mold toxicity. These nutrients support mitochondrial function, the powerhouse of the cell, and aid in the detoxification process. Focusing on a diet rich in antioxidants, healthy fats, and clean proteins can provide the necessary building blocks for recovery.

Antioxidants are crucial for combating oxidative stress, a condition exacerbated by mold exposure. Foods high in antioxidants include berries, leafy greens, nuts, and seeds. Berries, such as blueberries and raspberries, are not only rich in antioxidants but also contain vital vitamins and minerals that support energy levels and cognitive function. Leafy greens like spinach and kale are packed with vitamins A, C, and K, along with minerals such as iron and calcium, which are essential for energy production and detoxification.

Healthy fats, particularly omega-3 fatty acids, are vital for reducing inflammation and supporting brain health. Sources of omega-3s include fatty fish like salmon, chia seeds, flaxseeds, and walnuts. Incorporating these foods into your diet can help improve cognitive function and mood, both of which can be adversely affected by mold toxicity.

Clean proteins provide the amino acids necessary for repairing tissue and supporting the immune system. Opt for grass-fed, organic meats, and wild-caught fish to minimize exposure to toxins and pesticides. Plant-based proteins such as lentils, chickpeas, and quinoa are also excellent sources and can be especially beneficial for those with sensitivities to animal products.

Supplements can also play a supportive role in your recovery. Certain supplements are particularly beneficial for those recovering from mold toxicity:

- **Coenzyme Q10 (CoQ10)** enhances cellular energy production and has antioxidant properties.
- **Milk thistle** supports liver health and detoxification.
- **Magnesium** is critical for energy production and muscle function. Many individuals exposed to mold are found to be deficient in magnesium.
- **Vitamin D** is essential for immune function and mood regulation. Considering the potential for limited sun exposure during recovery, supplementation may be necessary.
- **B-complex vitamins** are vital for energy production and nervous system health. They play a key role in metabolizing proteins, fats, and carbohydrates into energy.

It's also important to stay **hydrated**. Proper hydration supports detoxification and energy levels. Aim for filtered water to minimize exposure to additional toxins. Adding lemon or lime can enhance the detoxifying effects and provide a boost of vitamin C.

Lastly, consider incorporating **fermented foods** into your diet to support gut health. Foods like sauerkraut, kimchi, and kefir are rich in probiotics, which can help restore the gut microbiome. A healthy gut is crucial for optimal detoxification, nutrient absorption, and immune function.

By focusing on these nutritional strategies, you can support your body's healing process, regain energy, and enhance your overall well-being as you recover from mold toxicity. Remember, individual needs may vary, so it's beneficial to work with a healthcare professional to tailor your diet and supplement regimen to your specific situation.

12.2: Gentle Exercise for Recovery

Incorporating gentle exercise into your recovery regimen can be transformative, offering both physical and mental benefits without overburdening your system. As you embark on this path, it's crucial to choose activities that align with your current health status and energy levels, gradually enhancing your strength and endurance. Here are specific low-impact exercises and movements designed to facilitate recovery, improve vitality, and ensure that you do not overextend yourself in the process.

Walking: Starting with short, leisurely walks can significantly boost your cardiovascular health, improve circulation, and elevate your mood. Initially, aim for a comfortable pace and distance that does not lead to fatigue. Gradually increase both as your endurance improves, listening to your body's signals to avoid overexertion.

Yoga: Yoga combines physical postures, breathing exercises, and meditation to enhance flexibility, strength, and mental clarity. Focus on gentle yoga styles, such as Hatha or restorative yoga, which are designed to be nurturing and accessible for beginners or those with health challenges. Yoga's emphasis on mindful movement and breath awareness can also be particularly beneficial for stress reduction.

Tai Chi: Often described as meditation in motion, Tai Chi is a gentle form of martial arts that involves slow, deliberate movements and deep breathing. This practice can improve balance, flexibility, and strength, making it an excellent choice for those recovering from mold toxicity. Tai Chi has also been shown to reduce stress and anxiety, contributing to emotional well-being.

Swimming and Water Aerobics: Water-based exercises are incredibly gentle on the joints and can be an excellent way to build strength and endurance. The buoyancy of water supports your body, reducing the risk of injury and strain. Swimming laps or participating in a water aerobics class can provide a comprehensive workout that is both refreshing and invigorating.

Pilates: Pilates focuses on core strength, flexibility, and mindful movement. Starting with basic mat exercises can help rebuild your strength, particularly in the core muscles, which are essential for overall stability and injury prevention. Pilates exercises can be easily modified to accommodate your fitness level and gradually become more challenging as your recovery progresses.

Stretching: Incorporating daily stretching routines can improve flexibility, reduce stiffness, and enhance circulation. Focus on gentle stretches that target major muscle groups, holding each stretch for 20-30 seconds without bouncing. Stretching is also an excellent opportunity to practice deep breathing, further promoting relaxation and stress relief.

Cycling: Stationary cycling or leisurely bike rides on flat terrain can be a great way to reintroduce aerobic exercise without high impact. Cycling helps build leg strength and endurance while being gentle on the joints. Ensure the bike is properly adjusted to your height to avoid strain, and start with shorter sessions, gradually increasing the duration as your fitness improves.

Gardening: Engaging in light gardening activities can be a therapeutic and gentle way to incorporate movement into your day. Activities like planting, weeding, and watering encourage gentle bending, stretching, and walking, providing a low-intensity workout. Additionally, spending time outdoors and connecting with nature can have a calming effect, enhancing mental health.

Dance: Dancing can be a joyful way to add gentle movement to your routine. Whether it's a structured dance class designed for beginners or simply moving to music at home, dancing can improve your mood, flexibility, and endurance. Choose styles that allow you to move at your own pace, focusing on the enjoyment of movement rather than intensity.

Incorporating these gentle exercises into your recovery process can significantly contribute to your physical and emotional healing. It's essential to start slowly, gradually increasing the intensity and duration of your activities as your strength and energy levels improve. Always consult with your healthcare provider before beginning any new exercise regimen, especially if you have specific health concerns or conditions. By mindfully integrating gentle movement into your daily routine, you can support your body's healing process, rebuild your energy and vitality, and enhance your overall well-being.

12.3: Sleep Optimization for Restful Nights

For individuals recovering from mold toxicity and chronic illness, optimizing sleep is a cornerstone of regaining energy and vitality. Sleep disturbances, including insomnia and unrestful sleep, can significantly hinder the body's ability to heal and rejuvenate. Here are targeted strategies to enhance sleep quality, tailored to address the unique challenges faced during recovery:

Create a Sleep-Conducive Environment: Your bedroom should be a sanctuary designed to promote restful sleep. Ensure your sleeping area is cool, dark, and quiet. Consider using blackout curtains to block out light, and a white noise machine or earplugs to drown out disruptive sounds. The ideal temperature for sleep is between 60-67 degrees Fahrenheit, as cooler environments tend to support better sleep.

Establish a Consistent Sleep Schedule: Going to bed and waking up at the same time every day, even on weekends, can significantly improve sleep quality. Consistency reinforces your body's sleep-wake cycle, making it easier to fall asleep and wake up naturally.

Limit Exposure to Blue Light: Exposure to blue light from screens (phones, tablets, computers, TVs) before bedtime can disrupt your natural sleep cycle. Try to avoid screen time at least one hour before going to sleep. If you must use these devices, consider using blue light filters or glasses that block blue light.

Mindful Consumption: Caffeine and alcohol can have profound effects on sleep quality. Avoid consuming caffeinated beverages late in the day and be mindful of alcohol intake, as it can lead to disrupted sleep patterns. Opt for calming herbal teas, such as chamomile or lavender, in the evening to promote relaxation.

Incorporate Relaxation Techniques: Engaging in relaxation techniques before bed can help ease the transition into sleep. Practices such as deep breathing exercises, progressive muscle relaxation, or guided imagery can reduce stress and anxiety, making it easier to fall asleep.

Optimize Your Bed for Comfort: Invest in a high-quality mattress and pillows that support your preferred sleeping position. The right bedding can make a significant difference in sleep quality. Additionally, ensure your bedding is made of breathable materials to keep you comfortable throughout the night.

Physical Activity: Regular, moderate exercise can improve sleep quality and help regulate sleep patterns. However, avoid vigorous exercise close to bedtime, as it can have the opposite effect and energize you. Gentle stretching or yoga in the evening can be beneficial.

Nutritional Support for Sleep: Certain foods can support better sleep. Foods rich in magnesium, such as almonds and spinach, and those high in tryptophan, like turkey and warm milk, can promote relaxation and aid in the production of sleep-inducing hormones.

Mind Your Sleep Position: Some sleep positions can exacerbate health issues, impacting sleep quality. For instance, sleeping on your back can worsen snoring and sleep apnea, while sleeping on your side can alleviate these issues. Experiment with different positions to find what works best for you.

Consider Professional Help: If sleep disturbances persist despite implementing these strategies, it may be beneficial to consult with a healthcare professional. They can help identify underlying issues contributing to poor sleep and recommend appropriate treatments, which may include cognitive-behavioral therapy for insomnia (CBT-I) or a tailored supplement regimen.

By adopting these strategies, you can create an optimal environment and routine that supports restful, restorative sleep. Remember, the journey to recovery from mold toxicity and chronic illness is multifaceted, and prioritizing sleep is a critical component of regaining your energy and vitality.

Chapter 13: Preventing Future Mold Exposure

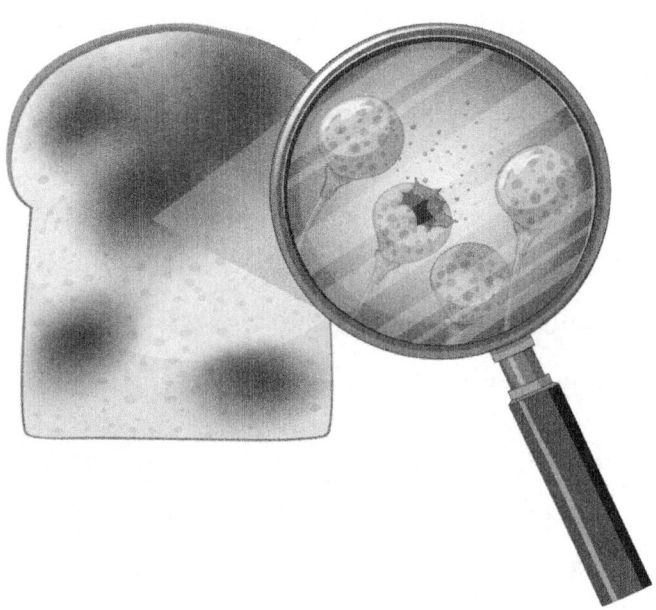

13.1: Identifying High-Risk Environments

In identifying high-risk environments for mold growth, it's crucial to understand that mold thrives in moist, warm, and poorly ventilated areas. Homes with poor insulation, water leaks, and inadequate ventilation are prime habitats for mold proliferation. Workplaces, especially older buildings with outdated HVAC systems, can also harbor mold in walls, ceilings, and air ducts. Climates with high humidity levels or regions prone to flooding are especially susceptible to mold issues.

To safeguard against mold exposure, start by inspecting areas where moisture accumulates. Look for visible signs of water damage, such as stains on walls or ceilings, which can indicate a conducive environment for mold growth. Bathrooms, kitchens, and basements are common areas where mold tends to manifest due to higher moisture levels.

Ensure these areas have adequate ventilation and use dehumidifiers in basements or other damp spaces to keep humidity levels below 50%.

In workplaces, advocate for regular HVAC inspections to ensure systems are properly filtering air and maintaining low humidity levels. Encourage the use of air purifiers with HEPA filters to capture mold spores circulating in the air.

For those living in humid climates, it's vital to maintain a vigilant approach to moisture control. After heavy rainfalls or floods, inspect your home for any water intrusion and address it promptly to prevent mold growth. Simple measures, such as cleaning gutters regularly and ensuring the ground slopes away from your home's foundation, can significantly reduce the risk of water damage and subsequent mold issues.

Materials used in construction can also impact mold growth. Opt for mold-resistant products when building or renovating your home. These products, including drywall and paints, contain mold inhibitors that help prevent mold from taking hold.

Regular home inspections are a proactive measure to identify potential mold issues early. Pay special attention to windows, roofs, and pipes for any signs of leaks or condensation. Addressing these issues promptly can prevent mold from becoming a larger problem.

In summary, identifying high-risk environments for mold growth involves a combination of vigilance, regular maintenance, and proactive moisture control measures. By understanding the conditions that favor mold growth and taking steps to mitigate these factors, individuals can significantly reduce their risk of mold exposure and protect their health and well-being.

13.2: Building a Mold-Resistant Home

When considering the construction or renovation of a home to make it resistant to mold, it's essential to focus on materials, techniques, and maintenance practices that minimize the risk of mold growth. Utilizing mold-resistant materials in your home's construction can significantly reduce the likelihood of mold development, even in areas prone to moisture. For instance, drywall designed to resist moisture absorption is a superior choice for bathrooms, kitchens, and basements where humidity levels are typically higher. Similarly, mold-resistant paint contains additives that prevent mold from growing on painted surfaces, offering an additional layer of protection in moisture-prone areas.

In terms of construction techniques, proper insulation and ventilation are crucial. Ensure that your home is well-insulated to prevent condensation, which can occur when warm, moist air meets cold surfaces, creating an ideal environment for mold growth. Proper ventilation, particularly in areas like the attic and basement, helps to regulate moisture levels within the home. Installing exhaust fans in bathrooms and kitchens can also expel moisture-laden air directly outside, preventing it from circulating throughout the house.

Maintenance practices play a vital role in keeping a home mold-resistant. Regularly inspecting and cleaning gutters and downspouts to ensure water is effectively diverted away from the home's foundation can prevent moisture accumulation that could lead to mold. Additionally, promptly repairing leaks in roofs, windows, and pipes reduces moisture entry points. Keeping indoor humidity levels below 50% by using dehumidifiers or air conditioners during humid months is another effective strategy to hinder mold growth.

Choosing flooring materials that resist moisture, such as tile or vinyl, can also aid in preventing mold in areas where spills or moisture are common. Carpets, which can trap moisture and provide a breeding ground for mold spores, should be avoided in basements, bathrooms, and kitchens.

Incorporating mold-resistant materials and construction techniques, coupled with diligent maintenance, can significantly mitigate the risk of mold growth in your home, safeguarding the health and well-being of its occupants. Regularly monitoring moisture levels and addressing any signs of mold early can ensure that your home remains a safe, mold-resistant environment.

13.3: Lifestyle Habits for Long-Term Health

Adopting daily practices that promote a mold-resistant lifestyle is essential for long-term health and vitality. These habits not only contribute to a healthier living environment but also support your body's resilience against potential mold exposure. Here are practical steps you can integrate into your daily routine:

1. **Maintain Proper Ventilation**: Ensure your living spaces are well-ventilated to prevent the accumulation of moisture, which fosters mold growth. Regularly open windows to allow fresh air circulation, especially in areas like the kitchen and bathroom where moisture levels are higher. Utilize exhaust fans to expel moisture-laden air directly outside.

2. **Control Humidity Levels**: Keeping indoor humidity levels in check is crucial. Use a hygrometer to monitor the humidity, aiming to keep it below 50%. Dehumidifiers can be particularly effective in damp areas of your home, such as basements, to maintain optimal humidity levels.

3. **Regular Home Inspections**: Conduct routine inspections of your home to identify potential mold hotspots. Pay close attention to windows, roofs, and plumbing for any signs of leaks or condensation. Early detection and remediation of moisture issues can prevent mold from taking root.

4. **Use Mold-Resistant Products**: When renovating or decorating your home, choose mold-resistant paints, drywall, and flooring materials. These products are designed to withstand moisture and can significantly reduce the risk of mold development.

5. **Implement Moisture Control Measures**: Simple actions like using a squeegee to remove excess water from shower walls, fixing leaky faucets promptly, and ensuring that the ground outside slopes away from your home's foundation can have a profound impact on moisture control.

6. **Optimize Air Quality**: Incorporate air-purifying plants into your home decor and consider using air purifiers with HEPA filters to capture mold spores and other allergens.

Regularly replace HVAC filters to ensure your system is effectively removing contaminants from the air.

7. **Embrace a Mold-Detoxifying Diet**: Incorporate foods that support detoxification and immune health, such as leafy greens, garlic, onions, and probiotics. Staying hydrated and limiting intake of sugar and processed foods can also bolster your body's defenses against mold.

8. **Stay Informed**: Educate yourself about mold, its health impacts, and prevention strategies. Knowledge is power, and staying informed enables you to make healthier choices for your living environment.

9. **Build a Support Network**: Connect with others who have experienced mold toxicity or are knowledgeable about mold prevention. Sharing experiences and tips can provide valuable insights and encouragement.

10. **Practice Stress-Reduction Techniques**: Chronic stress can weaken the immune system, making you more susceptible to mold-related health issues. Incorporate stress-reduction practices such as yoga, meditation, or deep-breathing exercises into your daily routine.

11. **Prioritize Sleep**: Quality sleep is essential for health and recovery. Ensure your bedroom is a mold-free sanctuary, and adopt sleep hygiene practices such as maintaining a regular sleep schedule and creating a restful environment.

12. **Stay Active**: Regular, gentle exercise can support detoxification processes and boost overall health. Choose activities you enjoy and that match your energy levels, such as walking, swimming, or tai chi.

By integrating these habits into your daily life, you can create a healthier, mold-resistant environment that supports your well-being and vitality. Remember, consistency is key. Making small, manageable changes over time can lead to significant improvements in your health and environment.

Resources and Appendices

Appendix A: DIY Mold Testing Checklist

1. **Gather Your Tools**: Before beginning, ensure you have the necessary equipment for DIY mold testing. This includes a digital humidity meter, flashlight, gloves, protective mask, and a mold testing kit available from most hardware stores. For remediation, gather cleaning supplies such as white vinegar, hydrogen peroxide, or a mold removal product certified by the Environmental Protection Agency (EPA), along with scrub brushes and plastic sheeting to contain the area.

2. **Check Humidity Levels**: Use your digital humidity meter to measure the humidity in various rooms. Mold thrives in environments with humidity levels above 60%, so identifying and addressing high humidity areas is crucial. If any room measures above this threshold, consider using a dehumidifier to reduce moisture.

3. **Visual Inspection**: With your flashlight, inspect dark and damp areas of your home, such as basements, attics, under sinks, and around windows. Look for visible signs of mold growth, which can range in color from black and green to white and orange. Pay special attention to water stains or discoloration on walls, ceilings, and floors, as these can indicate hidden mold.

4. **Use a DIY Mold Testing Kit**: Follow the instructions on your mold testing kit to collect samples from suspected areas. These kits typically involve taking surface samples with a swab or capturing airborne spores on a petri dish. After collecting samples, you'll either observe the growth of mold on the medium provided (for petri dish tests) or send the samples to a lab for analysis, depending on the kit's design.

5. **Interpreting Results**: If your DIY testing kit indicates the presence of mold or if you visually identify mold growth, it's time to plan your remediation strategy. For small, contained areas (less than 10 square feet), you may be able to handle the cleanup yourself. Larger infestations or mold in HVAC systems should be addressed by professionals.

6. **Prepare the Area**: Before beginning remediation, isolate the affected area to prevent the spread of spores. Use plastic sheeting to seal off the space and ensure you wear protective gear, including gloves, a mask, and eye protection.

7. **Remove Mold**: For non-porous surfaces like tile or metal, use a scrub brush and your chosen cleaning solution to remove the mold. For porous materials like drywall or carpet, you may need to cut out and dispose of the moldy material. Always follow the cleaning product's instructions for safe use.

8. **Dry the Area Thoroughly**: After cleaning, it's essential to dry the area completely to prevent mold from returning. Use fans or dehumidifiers to aid in drying out the space. Keep the area dry and monitor for any signs of mold returning in the following weeks.

9. **Prevent Future Growth**: Address the underlying moisture problem that led to mold growth. This may involve repairing leaks, improving ventilation, or using a dehumidifier regularly. Repaint cleaned areas with mold-resistant paint to provide an extra layer of protection against future mold growth.

10. **Regular Monitoring**: Even after remediation, continue to monitor your home for signs of mold or moisture issues. Regularly check areas previously affected by mold, as well as any other potential problem areas, to catch any new growth early.

By following these steps, you can effectively identify and address mold issues in your home, creating a safer and healthier living environment. Remember, tackling mold growth early and addressing the root cause of moisture can prevent larger, more costly problems down the line.

Appendix B: Supplement and Herb Guide

Vitamin C: An essential antioxidant that supports the immune system and aids in detoxifying the body. Suggested dosage: 1,000 to 3,000 mg daily, in divided doses.

Milk Thistle: Known for its liver-protective qualities, milk thistle supports detox pathways. Standardized extract dosage: 100 to 300 mg, twice daily.

Glutathione: Often referred to as the body's "master antioxidant," it plays a crucial role in detoxification processes. For oral supplementation, liposomal glutathione is recommended for better absorption, with dosages ranging from 500 to 1,000 mg daily.

Activated Charcoal: Binds to toxins in the gut, helping to reduce the burden on the liver by preventing reabsorption. Dosage: 500 to 1,000 mg taken with a large glass of water, ideally 1-2 hours away from food and medication to avoid nutrient absorption issues.

Curcumin: The active compound in turmeric, curcumin, offers powerful anti-inflammatory and detoxification support. Dosage: 500 to 1,000 mg of curcuminoids daily, often taken with piperine to enhance absorption.

Omega-3 Fatty Acids: Reduce inflammation and support cell membrane health, which is vital for detoxification and recovery. Dosage: 1,000 to 2,000 mg daily of EPA and DHA combined.

Probiotics: Essential for gut health, which is intrinsically linked to overall health and detoxification. Look for strains like Lactobacillus and Bifidobacterium. Dosage: 10 to 50 billion CFUs daily, taken with food.

N-acetylcysteine (NAC): Supports the production of glutathione and offers additional detoxification and antioxidant support. Dosage: 600 to 1,200 mg daily, in divided doses.

Dandelion Root: Acts as a diuretic to help flush toxins from the body and supports liver function. Dosage: 500 to 2,000 mg daily, in divided doses or as a tea.

Green Tea Extract: Contains catechins, powerful antioxidants that support detoxification. Dosage: 250 to 500 mg daily, standardized to contain 40 to 50 percent EGCG.

Chlorella: A green algae that binds to heavy metals and supports their elimination from the body. Dosage: 3,000 to 5,000 mg daily, taken in divided doses.

Spirulina: Another algae rich in proteins and antioxidants, supporting overall detoxification. Dosage: 3,000 to 5,000 mg daily, in divided doses.

Ashwagandha: An adaptogen that helps the body manage stress, which is crucial for recovery and detoxification. Dosage: 300 to 500 mg daily of an extract standardized to contain 5% withanolides.

Ginger: Offers gastrointestinal support, aiding in the elimination of toxins. Can be taken as a supplement or used fresh. Dosage for supplements: 500 to 1,000 mg daily.

Garlic: Known for its immune-boosting and detoxification support. Allicin is the active component, so look for products standardized to contain a certain amount of allicin. Dosage: 600 to 1,200 mg daily, in divided doses.

Zinc: Supports immune function and has a protective effect against heavy metal toxicity. Dosage: 15 to 30 mg daily, taken with food to avoid stomach upset.

Selenium: An antioxidant that helps protect the body from heavy metals and supports thyroid function. Dosage: 100 to 200 mcg daily.

Magnesium: Essential for hundreds of biochemical reactions in the body, including detoxification processes. Dosage: 200 to 400 mg daily, preferably in the form of magnesium glycinate for better absorption and gastrointestinal tolerance.

This guide is designed to provide a starting point for those looking to support their body's detoxification and recovery processes through supplementation. It's important to consult with a healthcare provider before starting any new supplement regimen, especially for individuals with existing health conditions or those taking medication, to ensure safety and appropriateness.

Printed in Dunstable, United Kingdom